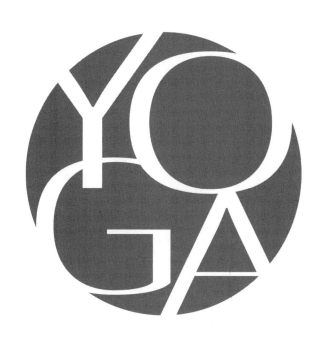

Some of the postures contained in this publication should only be attempted under the supervision of an experienced yoga practitioner. If in doubt, please contact your doctor or local yoga center.

Published by:
Ulysses Press
P.O. Box 3440
Berkeley CA 94703
www.ulyssespress.com

Library of Congress Control Number 2003104411
ISBN 1-56975-366-0

First published by HarperCollins Publishers, Sydney, Australia, in 2001.
This edition published by arrangement with HarperCollins Publishers Pty Ltd.

Printed in Canada by Transcontinental Printing

1 3 5 7 9 10 8 6 4 2

Cover model: Jessie Chapman
All photographs by Dhyan

Yoga models: James Bahuth, Jessie Chapman, Mark Hill, Rachel Hull, Peter Watkins

JESSIE CHAPMAN

photographs by
DHYAN

YOGA

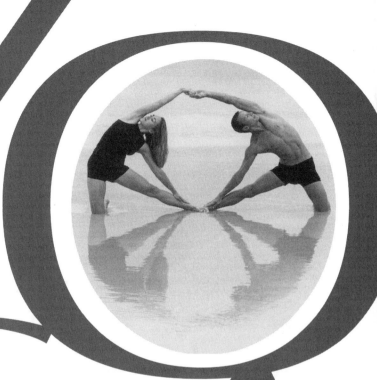

THERAPIES

45 Sequences to relieve stress, depression,
repetitive strain, sports injuries and more

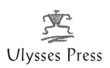

Ulysses Press

Contents

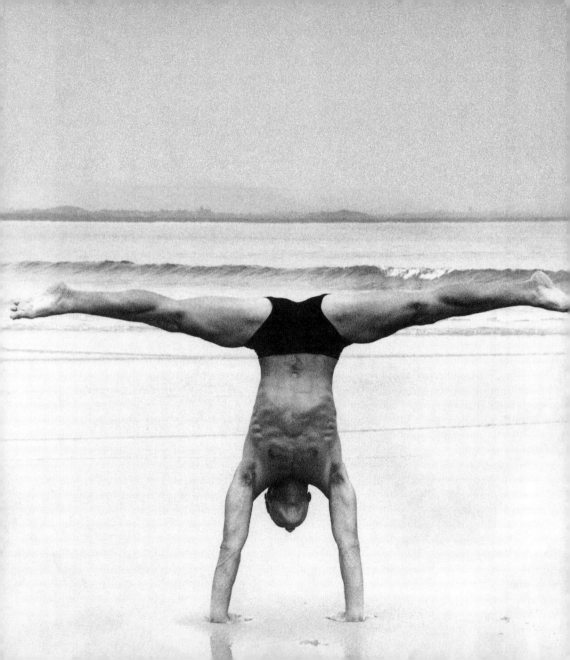

Insight into yoga

The origins of yoga

Ancient yogis observed and studied nature, life's cycles and people to create a system that brought balance to one's mental and emotional states and physical body, freeing one's spirit and realizing a way of living in true happiness and wholeness of being.

Most of us experience moments of wholeness, and in those times, we often feel totally at peace with ourselves, others and life.

The practices or disciplines of yoga draw our attention inward, to a place of stillness, where self-realization or wholeness, the ultimate goal of yoga practice, is realized.

Yoga is just one branch of ancient India's family tree of philosophical traditions. The different branches of this tree of life are recorded in the *Book of Vedas*. These and other holy scriptures were originally written in Sanskrit, a language that was only used and understood by the educated few, higher caste members and priests.

Since the philosophy of yoga and the details of its practice were recorded in a sacred language, they were for a long time inaccessible to the masses, many of whom could not read. But, eventually, as interest in yoga grew and more people applied themselves to its study, the understanding of the philosophy increased until, in around 300 BC, Patanjali, a great Indian sage known as the "father of yoga," helped overcome the language barrier by translating the philosophy into a common language. Known as the *yoga sutras*, Patanjali's bite-sized phrases illuminated the path for millions of people in the future to find and practice yoga. Within the *sutras*, Patanjali systemized – and thereby helped demystify – the practice and discipline of yoga into an eightfold path known as the "eight limbs of yoga." Patanjali was able to weave together this ancient philosophy, revealing a path that could free one from negative beliefs, limiting lifestyle habits and give us the tools to discover our highest potential in life.

The Sanskrit word for yoga is *yuj*, meaning to unite, bind or yoke. And over time, it became widely practiced by many, reflecting the essence of yoga in its own name, that of togetherness and oneness.

As its popularity as a spiritual path exploded throughout India, the number of yoga teachers (gurus), ashrams (retreats or communities where a Hindu holy man lives) and disciples grew. Eventually, travelers from around the world discovered yoga and brought it, along with the Eastern way of life, to the West.

Yoga illuminated

The complete eight limb yoga system, as developed by Patanjali, includes many yoga practices such as *asanas* (physical postures) and *pranayama* (regulated breathing), taught in most Hatha yoga classes.

This eightfold path helped illuminate the philosophy behind yoga and made it accessible to people seeking to get in touch with themselves and a spiritual path. Each limb, or discipline, is a part of the complete yoga system. These mental and physical disciplines were designed to be integrated and practiced as a whole rather than in separate parts, promoting a balanced way of life.

The eight limbs of yoga

1. YAMAS
Guides for us to live in harmony with one another in a shared and peaceful world.

2. NIYAMAS
Personal disciplines that relate to the body and mind. They include cleanliness of mind, body and environment; contentment; practice or dedication; personal growth and inspiration; and study of the self.

3. ASANA
Physical postures designed to cleanse, stretch and strengthen the body in preparation for sitting in meditation and to develop self-awareness.

4. PRANAYAMA
Regulated breathing techniques that teach us to breathe fully and correctly, increasing our intake and absorption of *prana*, or life force, and our energy levels.

5. PRATYAHARA

Removal of the self from the search for constant stimulation and satisfaction in the world, turning the focus inward to experience silence and peace within yourself.

6. DHARANA

The practice of concentration that leads to calmness of the mind. With practice, entering a quiet, meditative space becomes more effortless and more desirable.

7. DHYANA

Meditation. Through meditation we experience the mind emptying itself of thoughts and desires. The whole being benefits from this "time out."

8. SAMADHI

A state of being total, united and present in the moment. Known as enlightenment or self-realization, this is the ultimate spiritual goal of yoga practice.

Yoga paths

There are many different paths of yoga, each making up an important aspect of yoga philosophy as a whole.

Hatha yoga is one of the most common forms of yoga practiced in the West. Being a yoga of force or technique, it includes *asanas* (the physical postures) and *pranayama* (the regulated breathing techniques) to promote a healthy, balanced mind and body.

The word Hatha combines *ha* (sun) and *tha* (moon), representing unison of the opposite forces and elements at play in our body and in life. *Pranayama* and *asana* practice makes *dhyana* (meditation or sitting in stillness) more comfortable as the body is made more flexible and the mind quieter.

Other yoga paths involve different practices. *Jnana* yoga, the yoga of knowledge, self-study and learning, involves studying the holy scriptures and absorbing teachings through the written word. *Bhakti* yoga is a path of devotion, where all one's thoughts and actions become a service offered to a higher cause or source. *Karma* yoga, the yoga of service, is where one's work is offered without expectation of reward or gratification.

Different people are drawn to different aspects of yoga, but with regular practice we become attuned to its other aspects, deepening our understanding of its philosophy. Today, many of the different yoga paths can be learned in classes. Check with your local yoga school or society to see what's available.

Yoga is evolving

As humans continue living at a fast pace and technology keeps progressing, the number of people turning within to find peace and a spiritual connection is growing rapidly. Being a nonjudgmental path, yoga practice has likewise seen a rapid growth, with yoga schools, centers, ashrams and teachers dedicated to its various forms now abundant worldwide.

Traditionally, yoga was taught one on one. The teacher would administer yoga postures specific to the individual's needs and conditions. Since yoga's popularity has increased, the yoga class has evolved to accommodate many different people at the same time, as well as different styles of yoga. Whether practicing yoga alone, one on one, or in a large group, self-awareness remains the key to receiving yoga as a therapy to mind and body.

Changing times, different environments and the diverse backgrounds and ideologies of its teachers have seen yoga evolve into many styles. However, because of yoga's essential essence being as powerful as it is, its ability to connect people to themselves, each other, to nature, life, love and wisdom, has remained strong and unchanging throughout time.

One of the greatest attractions of yoga is its all-embracing quality – of cultures, beliefs and religions. It remains an open path without dogma, its main concern being to develop a healthy mind and body. No matter what type of lifestyle you lead or other paths you follow, a connection with yoga can be found within.

Yoga and you

With the practice of the yoga postures, breathing and meditation, you get to know your body and your self. Yoga develops self-awareness. As you learn about your self, you will discover new talents, skills, dreams and passions, making your life richer.

Your yoga practice is a time to stop, relax, connect within; grow, expand, change; and become strong and flexible. It is a time to be still and listen to your inner voice and develop self-awareness.

Just as each day is new and offers a fresh beginning, each yoga practice offers changing experiences. Your yoga journey is a personal path, as well as a path of connecting with the whole; going within we experience more understanding and connection with the world and others.

Explore your self through yoga practice. Find a teacher and a style of yoga you connect with, trust and can learn from. A good teacher will help you to develop awareness and to become your own teacher. Since no one knows your body or your self better than you do, it makes sense to deepen your understanding of your self and discover inner wisdom.

Working in the postures

Asana, Sanskrit for "posture," also translates as "to be." "Being" in *asana* we experience and learn the essence of yoga, that of unity. Your physical self, your breath and your intention are united when you become present and grounded in your body.

Through regular dedicated practice, your ability to perform the postures develops and all aspects of your self are united to create balance and a feeling of wholeness.

Awareness is the key to understanding yoga through the physical postures. Patanjali describes the practice of the postures as a balance between *sthira* and *sukha*, or alertness and lightness, action and relaxation. Balancing these qualities consciously, the posture comes alive and is energized without straining or pushing.

Finding a balance between wanting to go further in the pose and accepting where the body is in the pose, you allow the essence of yoga to touch you. Whether you let go completely, or activate, open or hold, soften or contract, the more you practice, the more tuned in you become to the desired action or non-action and outcome.

Mind-body connection

The practice of yoga affects us on all levels, bringing about a union of the body, mind and spirit; with continued practice, the mind, body and spirit all become more open, strong and flexible. And just as during a yoga posture, our body is flexed, as is our open-mindedness. During meditation, the mind − as well as the emotions and physical body − is calmed. This interconnectedness that is a part of the yoga journey is constant and leads to the development of self-awareness and a deeper understanding of the nature of life.

People who have practiced yoga consistently throughout their lives speak about how it has brought more awareness, clarity, knowledge and wisdom; more harmony in their relationships, business and play; and the profound experience of knowing themselves. In physical terms, they speak of more strength and flexibility, and of an increased sense of aliveness and vitality in the whole body.

Effects on all levels

Yoga postures work intelligently with the body to bring all aspects of our self into a healthy and balanced state. Each body, or individual, is affected differently, according to his or her needs. Whichever part or area is overused will be relaxed, and whatever is underused will be stimulated.

Postures stimulate the nervous system, glands, digestion, circulation and organ function of your system if it is sluggish, or they will relax you if you are feeling overworked.

Different postures challenge us in different ways. Those requiring strength and balance encourage us to get in touch with our inner strength as we strive to perform the posture fully and correctly. In this process our willpower develops and our mind is cleansed, promoting clarity of thought and intention. Postures requiring flexibility challenge us to become soft and open, to let go of any holding on in the body and any limitations of the mind.

Mentally, we are also softened and strengthened into harmonious balance. Hard-headed, uptight and stressed people will have their overactive minds opened and relaxed. Lazy, dull minds are activated to become more alert and focused, and their owners will become clear-headed.

Through the practice of yoga, we become more in tune with our emotions; we learn when to listen to them or when to move on. Highly emotional people experience a shift away from the emotional state being the center of importance. People with blocked emotions who hold their feelings in and find it hard to express themselves experience greater understanding of themselves and of their connection to the whole, which allows for release of fear and open expression.

Releasing and letting go

We constantly need to let go in our everyday lives, and sometimes this can be very difficult or even painful to do. Yoga practice teaches us and gives us the tools to let go. Developing this ability to let go builds inner strength and helps relieve suffering.

When we practice yoga, letting go happens on all levels: we let go of any holding on in our body, we let go of thinking and thoughts in our mind, and we let go of focusing on our emotions.

The breath is a major tool in letting go. In a posture, we relax the muscles when we focus on softening with the exhalation. To quiet the mind of thoughts we focus on the sound of the breath, and keep returning to this focal point whenever we find ourselves wandering off to think again. When we experience strong and distracting emotions, we can utilize deep, full breathing to help release them.

By opening up, releasing and letting go in the mind and body, our spirit is renewed, re-energized and set free!

Practicing the sequences

Yoga practiced at sunrise or sunset is ideal. At sunrise we are in tune with the forces of nature; we can rise and stretch to the new day and feel renewed and at peace within. At dusk we wind down with the setting sun, turning inward and preparing for the night. However, due to our different lifestyles and work commitments, finding a suitable time to practice may mean attending a class during a lunchbreak or in the evening after work.

The yoga space

An open heart, pure intention and physical action are all that is really required to create a harmonious yoga space. Finding a place where you feel peaceful, away from everyday distractions, also helps you to get in the mood for yoga – a setting with quiet surroundings is ideal. If a tranquil setting is not available, then allow the simplicity of the breath and your position on the floor available, your sacred space.

When sharing a practice, the combined energies of the group make for an inspiring yoga space. If practicing alone, be creative – your yoga space could be the floor of your living room, or a flat surface under a tree in a garden or park.

A yoga mat or rug is good to practice yoga on and makes for a handy yoga space when traveling. A hard, flat surface is good for balance and focus in the postures.

But always remember, the practice itself is the important part and is all the yoga space you need.

Clothing and equipment

If you're practicing in a warm climate, you can simply wear cotton underwear. In colder climates, wear long-sleeved tops and long pants to keep the body warm and to help get heat circulating. Have a slightly lighter layer underneath so that you can strip off if necessary.

Cool, natural fibers are best; they allow the body to breathe and don't release chemicals that may be absorbed by the skin.

Yoga is practiced barefoot to allow for maximum circulation and contact with the floor.

Be prepared for *Savasana* or relaxation. Because the body cools down quickly when we stop to rest, have a warm layer of clothing on hand or a sarong ready to cover your body with, as well as an eye bag to relax the eyes, and socks to keep the feet warm in cooler climates.

In the privacy of your own home, try practicing yoga naked for a completely unrestricted and free feeling.

If you do not have "official" yoga props, many household items can be used in their place. Blocks are helpful for the standing postures – if you can't reach the floor, place a hand on a block or pile of books. Straps, or a belt, are helpful for extending into the forward bending postures. Bolsters or cushions are great to lie over to open the chest and assist in deep, full breathing, and blankets make good props and support in many *asanas*.

Warming up and winding down

Before practicing the yoga sequences, it's important to warm up. Getting heat circulating throughout the body, and especially the muscles, prevents soft tissue injury in the stretching postures. Warmed up, we experience the fullness of the pose and the richness of its benefits.

The general sequences in Chapter 6 include five warm-up practices: the dynamic salutes (*Surya Namaskar*), gentle warm-ups such as the East-West sequence, and Cat Curls. Choose one of these sequences to practice as a warm-up before the Remedial, Body, Sports, and Emotions and Moods sequences.

Just as important as warming up is allowing time to relax after practicing the yoga sequences. Sitting quietly, breathing, meditating and lying in *Savasana* all help to create a well-rested and balanced outcome. Yoga postures stimulate energies throughout the body, which are then able to settle and relax with winding-down postures and techniques. People who don't allow time to relax after yoga practice may feel "wired" and unsettled, especially if their practice has included dynamic postures.

After stretching and exercising the body, it actually becomes easier to focus on breathing and sit quietly in meditation – the higher aim of yoga practice. In this quiet space, we can become aware of the yoga experience, rich and powerful effects that include calmness of mind and a relaxed body.

To wind down at the end of the sequences, practice relaxing postures such as *Salamba Sarvangasana*, and spend time breathing or in meditation and *Savasana*.

Precautions and contraindications

Keep your yoga practice safe by listening to your body and communicating freely with your yoga instructor. Combining your intuition with the teacher's knowledge and experience will help to avoid injuries from overstretching or the practice of postures unsuitable for certain conditions.

Women are commonly instructed to avoid all inverted and dynamic postures when menstruating, and during pregnancy to practice only postures that don't constrict breathing or the baby's positioning in any way. Consult a yoga teacher for advice on safe yoga practice during pregnancy; there are numerous postures recommended for the optimum health and well-being of your baby and yourself.

If you have any known or suspected medical problems, always communicate them to your teacher. A qualified remedial yoga teacher can give you postures to aid in the resolution and relief of certain ailments and diseases, and will advise which postures to avoid in particular illnesses and physical problems. If uncertain, consult a medical doctor.

When you're exhausted, it's best to practice only passive postures that restore the body's energy levels. Wait two to three hours after eating before practicing yoga. If any postures feel "wrong," release out of them slowly with the breath. No one knows your body better than you do, so get into the habit of listening within for the best advice.

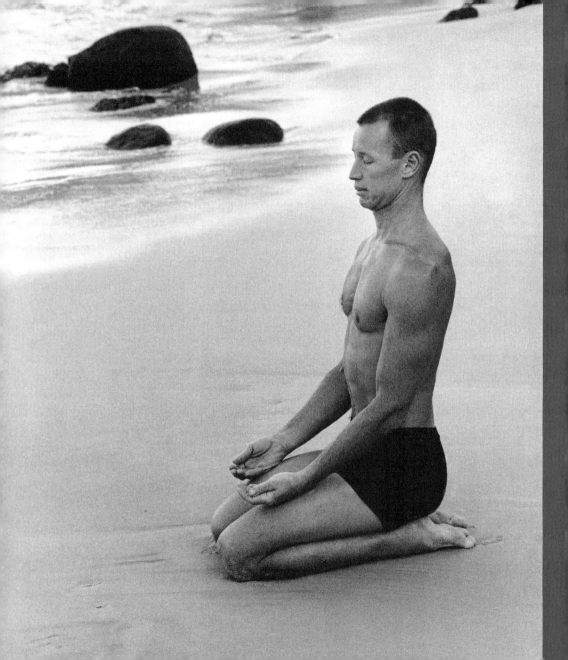

Breath focus

re breathing fully, taking in lots of fresh air, and cleansing the blood and wastes, we feel renewed and inspired. "Inspire" literally means "to breathe in." Freely circulating oxygen through the body is an energy charge, giving us more "get up and go," and "kick in our heels." The brain also thrives on fresh air and when well-oxygenated makes us feel creative, alert, clear and inspired.

Good health and fresh air go hand in hand. People often comment on how inspired they feel when surrounded by nature, and how healthy their skin looks and glows – that's one of the by-products of a well-oxygenated body.

Many people, rushing through life carrying tension and stress, never breathe fully or correctly. With constricted lungs, tight chest muscles and hunched shoulders, the flow of air – oxygen – is blocked. Apart from making you feel dull and lethargic, shallow and constricted breathing can lead to health-related problems such as hypertension and depression.

Being clear-headed is associated with being well-oxygenated, and both, therefore, help to clear the mind of busy thoughts and release stress from the body – giving a new perspective on life.

One of the main aspects of yoga practice is *pranayama*, which teaches us to breathe through the nose, to lengthen and deepen our breath, and increase our lung capacity and our life force. *Prana* means "life force," *yama* means "control." The vital life force *prana* is taken in with the breath.

Clear the mind, get inspired and be healthy – all through the yoga breath!

Inspiring for inspiration

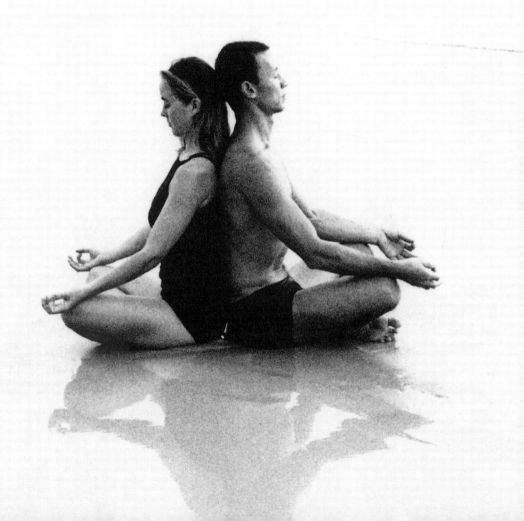

Deep, full breathing

Positioning: Sit in a comfortable position (see sitting positions in Chapter 3) resting the back of the hands on the knees. Softly close the eyes and focus on sitting correctly. Bring your spine into an upright position, roll the shoulders down and back to open the chest. For the breath to fill the lungs completely, it must reach the bottom, middle and top lobes of the lungs.

Technique: As you inhale through your nose, your abdomen draws in and moves back slightly toward the spine, the diaphragm inflates and the chest rises. The right and left rib cages move out to the sides and the collarbones lift. The inflowing breath is smooth and rhythmic. On exhaling, the diaphragm deflates and lowers as the air flows out softly and evenly.

Focus: On the soft sound of your breath as you inhale and exhale. Keep your spine straight in an upright position and the chest lifted.

Hold: Repeat for 10 full breaths, or longer if it's comfortable.

Benefits: This posture purifies the blood, and oxygenates and energizes the body and mind. It stimulates the brain, calms the nervous system, releases stress and helps to prevent many illnesses and diseases.

Precautions: Stop practicing if you experience tightness in the chest or shortness of breath, or if you start feeling anxious. Its purpose is to relax and calm the mind and body.

With maximum intake of oxygen to the lungs and maximum expulsion of wastes, correct breathing promotes relaxation and a healthy, disease-free body.

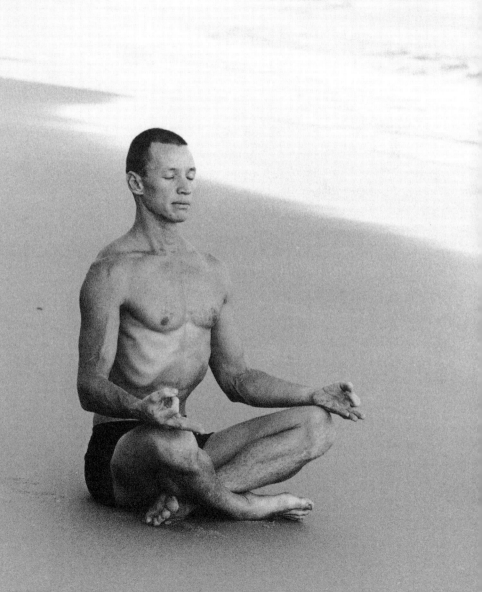

Alternate-nostril breathing

Positioning: Sit in a comfortable position (see sitting positions in Chapter 3). Make sure your spine is straight and your head is facing forward. Raise your right arm, bringing the palm of your hand toward your nose. Bend the index and second fingers and tuck them behind the thumb. The little finger and the ring finger remain extended.

Technique: Exhale fully and then lightly close the left nostril with gentle pressure from the extended ring and small fingers; inhale fully through the right nostril. Close the right nostril with the thumb, release the pressure on the left nostril and exhale fully through the left nostril. Inhale fully through the left nostril, close the left and open the right nostril. Exhale fully through the right nostril. This is one complete cycle.

Focus: Keep the breath flowing evenly through the right and left nostrils. Apply light pressure to the closed nostril. Keep your spine straight, and your head and right arm lifted and facing forward. Relax your head, neck and shoulders.

Hold: Repeat for 10 full cycles, or for as long as is comfortable.

Benefits: Clears the nasal passages and calms the mind. Develops willpower and self-awareness as you draw your attention inward.

Precautions: Stop practicing if you experience tightness in the chest or shortness of breath, or if you start to feel anxious. Its purpose is to relax and calm the mind and body.

The gentle inhalation and exhalation through alternate nostrils has a soothing and balancing effect, calming the nervous system and the mind.

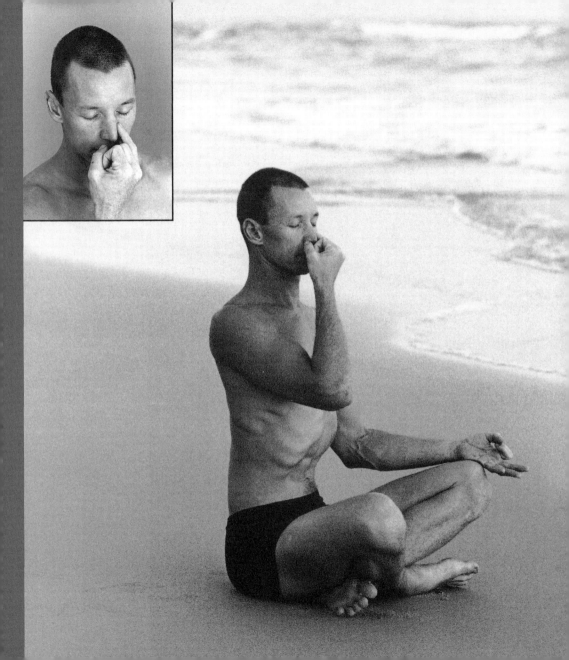

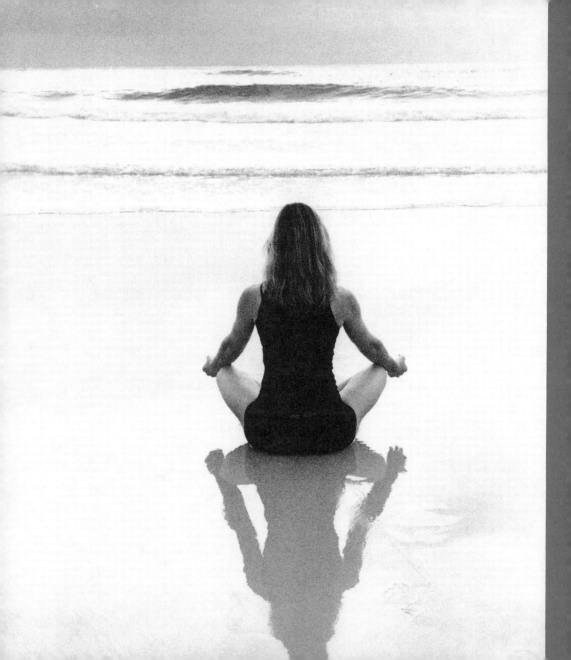

Meditation

The practice of meditation involves making a personal choice to turn your focus inward to a quiet, inner space of stillness. Practicing this drawing inward develops your ability to control your mind's chatter and allows your self-awareness to grow so that you are more able to make choices in life that lead to inner happiness and peace of mind.

Sitting in stillness teaches that being is often better than doing. Each day we are challenged by society, and ourselves, to do, to be, and to become more. However, allowing time to stop working, playing or exercising and to simply sit in quietness enables us to experience an island of peace.

The many roles we have in our lives – be they mother, father, lover, daughter, son, employer or employee – are emptied from us, along with expectations and thoughts, as we enter an empty space within where we can find simplicity and happiness.

With meditation practice, we become more present in the moment; our ability to focus increases; we regain clarity of mind, a good memory and a calm nervous system; and we experience increased self-love.

Find a quiet place away from any distractions. Sit in a comfortable position with your spine straight and your head facing forward. The mind can be a challenge to quiet, but with consistent practice and focus it becomes easier and the experience becomes more rewarding.

Meditating in a group and with a teacher to guide you can be helpful. Check your local yoga school or service directory for class availability.

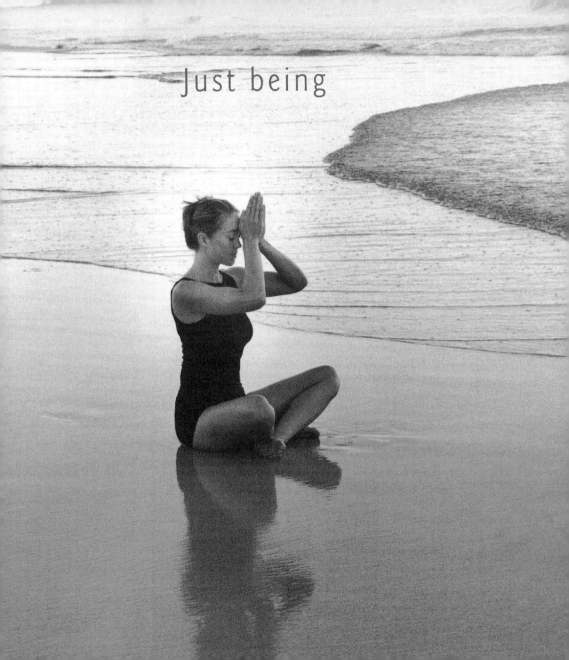

Just being

Virasana meditation

VIRA – A HERO

Positioning: Kneel, then sit with your knees bent and your buttocks resting on your heels. Draw your knees together and your feet together. Relax the back of your hands on your thighs, resting your shoulders and arms. Keep your spine straight and your head upright.

Breathing: Breathe softly through your nose.

Focus: Softly close your eyes and find a point of focus within your being to maintain while meditating. You can focus on the sound of your breathing, the gentle rise and fall of your chest, the air moving in and out of your nostrils, or on your third eye. When you find your mind wandering, return to your chosen point of focus.

Hold: For a few minutes or as long as comfortable. Extend your meditation time as you become more practiced.

Variations: Rest your legs and knees on one or more folded blankets to relieve tight ankles and feet. Put one or more folded blankets under your buttocks to relieve leg strain.

Benefits: Meditation practice gives you a vacation from your "mind stuff" and allows you to develop the ability to detach from emotional states. It promotes inner calm and refreshes the soul. The *Virasana* posture strengthens the pelvic muscles and knee and ankle joints, and stimulates digestion.

Sitting lightly, with no strain on the body, the mind is more able to relax and draw inward, away from the distractions of the world.

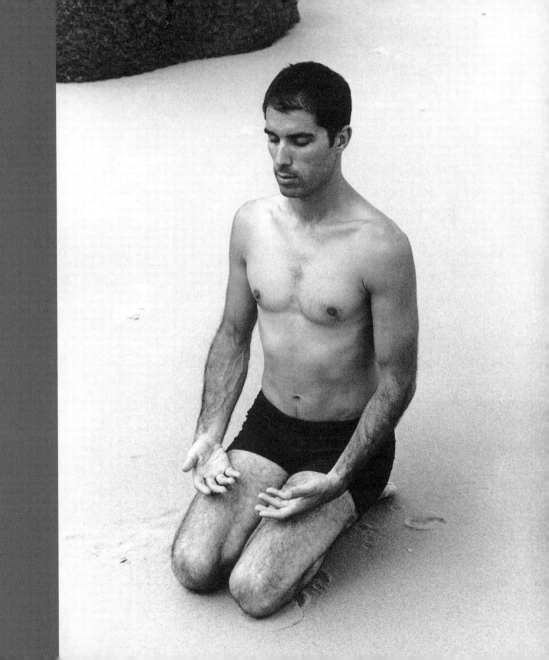

Siddhasana meditation

SIDDHA – SAGE OR SEMI-DIVINE BEING

Positioning: Sitting with your legs outstretched, bend your right leg and place the heel of the right foot into the groin. Next, bend your left leg and sit the heel of the left foot on top of the right heel, drawing it close into your pubis. Keep your spine, neck and head straight and in line. Rest the back of your hands on your knees. Bend the index finger of each hand and place it behind the thumbnail. Straighten the other three fingers out. This hand *mudra* (symbol) is called *Jnana* (knowledge); the action turns the nerve impulses inward to help deepen relaxation.

Breathing: Breathe softly and evenly through the nose.

Focus: Close your eyes and draw your focus inward to your third eye, the point between your eyebrows. Whenever you find your mind wandering, return your awareness to the third eye point of focus and let go of any thoughts.

Hold: For a few minutes or as long as comfortable. Extend your meditation time as you become more practiced.

Benefits: Meditation practice develops a sharp, clear and focused mind. It relaxes the nervous system, and helps develop self-awareness, self-love, confidence, intuition and a happy perspective on life. The *Siddhasana* posture flexes the hip and knee joints, and promotes good posture and a strong back.

This position promotes free-flowing *prana* through the spine and whole body. Feel yourself filling with life force.

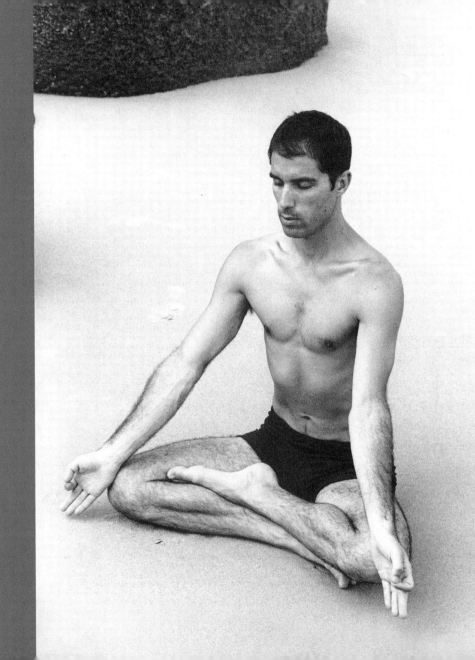

Sukhasana meditation

SUKHA - HAPPY

Positioning: Sit in an easy cross-legged position with the backs of your hands resting on your knees. Keep your spine straight and your head facing forward. Open your chest and soften your shoulders, rotating them back and down. Bend the index finger of each hand and place it behind the thumbnail. Straighten the other three fingers out. This hand *mudra* (symbol) is called *Jnana* (knowledge); the action turns the nerve impulses inward to help deepen relaxation.

Breathing: Breathe softly and evenly through the nose.

Focus: With eyes closed, turn your focus inward to the soft sound of the air flowing in and out of your nostrils. Maintain a point of focus to guide you into a space away from thinking, allowing your mind to empty of all thoughts.

Hold: For as long as comfortable. Start with a few minutes and lengthen with practice.

Variations: Sit with your buttocks on a folded blanket for support. Sit with your back resting against a wall for support, keeping your spine erect. Wrap a cloth gently around your head to cover your eyes, to help draw your attention inward. Wrap a cloth around your waist to help draw your lower back in and keep your spine straight.

Benefits: Sitting in stillness develops a sharp, clear and focused mind. It relaxes the nervous system, and helps develop self-awareness, self-love, confidence, intuition and a happy perspective on life. The *Sukhasana* position flexes the hip and knee joints, and promotes good posture and a strong back.

Being comfortable is imperative when practicing meditation. Reducing physical discomfort prevents the mind from wandering and makes it easier to meditate.

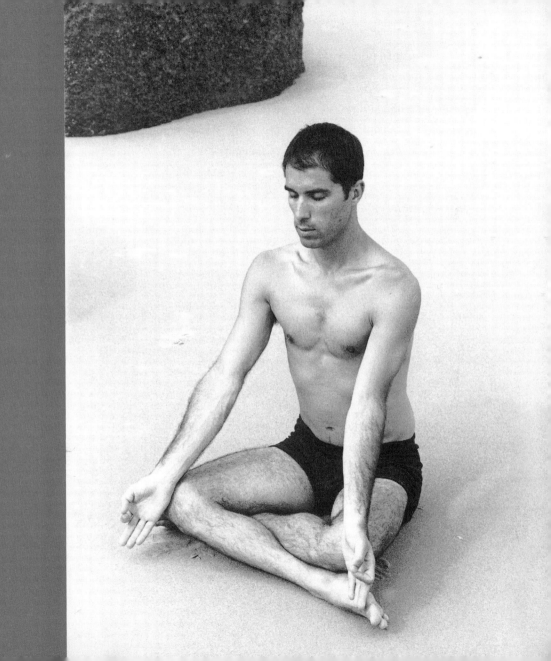

Ardha Padmasana meditation

ARDHA – HALF; PADMA – LOTUS

Positioning: Sit with your legs outstretched, then bend one leg and place the foot of that leg comfortably near the body. Bend your other leg, and raise the foot of that leg up onto the thigh of the opposite leg. Let your top knee release toward the floor as your hip softens. From this position, extend your upper body, lifting your chest and straightening your spine and head. Rest the backs of your hands on your knees, and bend the index finger of each hand and place it behind the thumbnail. Straighten the other three fingers out. This hand *mudra* (symbol) is called *Jnana* (knowledge); the action turns the nerve impulses inward to help deepen relaxation.

Breathing: Breathe softly and evenly through the nose.

Focus: Close your eyes and draw your focus inward to your third eye, the point between your eyebrows. Whenever you find your mind wandering, return your awareness to the third eye point of focus and let go of any thoughts.

Hold: For a few minutes or as long as comfortable. Extend your meditation time as you become more practiced.

Benefits: Meditation practice calms your mind, the nervous system and all the other body systems. The *Ardha Padmasana* posture loosens your hip and knee joints, helps develop a strong and healthy back, increases blood supply to your reproductive organs and relieves pelvic congestion.

34

The half lotus position is a **preparation** *asana* for full *Padmasana*. You may be limited to doing this position until your body loosens to allow the **full lotus**. Try alternating you leg positions to **stretch** both hips

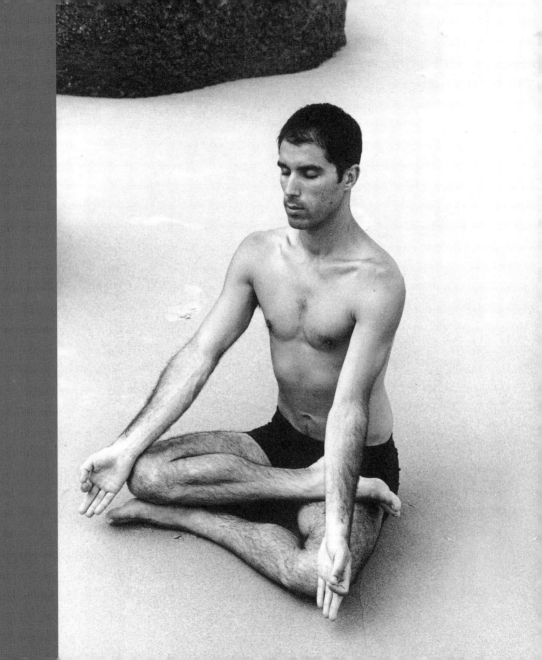

Padmasana meditation

Positioning: Sit with your legs outstretched and your buttocks on a folded blanket. Bend your right leg and bring the foot up onto your left thigh, with your right knee on the floor. Next, bend your left leg and bring the foot up onto the upper thigh of your right leg. Draw both feet as close as possible to your body and rest your knees on or toward the floor. Sit back into your sitting bones. With this firm lower body base, extend your upper body, lifting your chest and straightening your spine and head. Rest the backs of your hands on your knees. Bend the index finger of each hand and place it behind the thumbnail. Straighten the other three fingers out. This hand *mudra* (symbol) is called *Jnana* (knowledge); the action turns the nerve impulses inward to help deepen relaxation.

Breathing: Breathe softly and evenly through the nose.

Focus: Close your eyes and draw your focus inward to your third eye, the point between your eyebrows. Whenever you find your mind wandering, return your awareness to the third eye point of focus and let go of any thoughts.

Hold: For a few minutes or as long as comfortable. Extend your meditation time as you become more practiced.

Benefits: Meditation practice calms your mind, the nervous system and all other body systems. The *Padmasana* posture loosens your hip and knee joints, helps develop a strong and healthy back, increases blood supply to your reproductive organs and relieves pelvic congestion.

The unfolding beauty of the lotus flower symbolizes humankind's spiritual awakening. This position is ideal for meditative sitting, as it helps the mind ascend to a higher realm of inner calm.

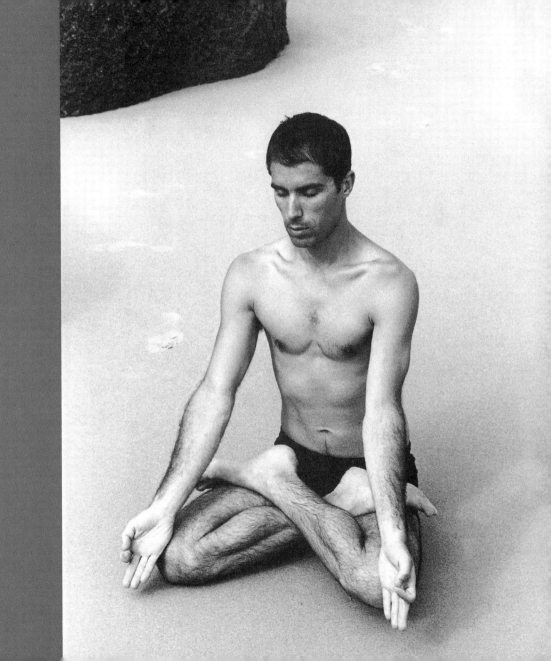

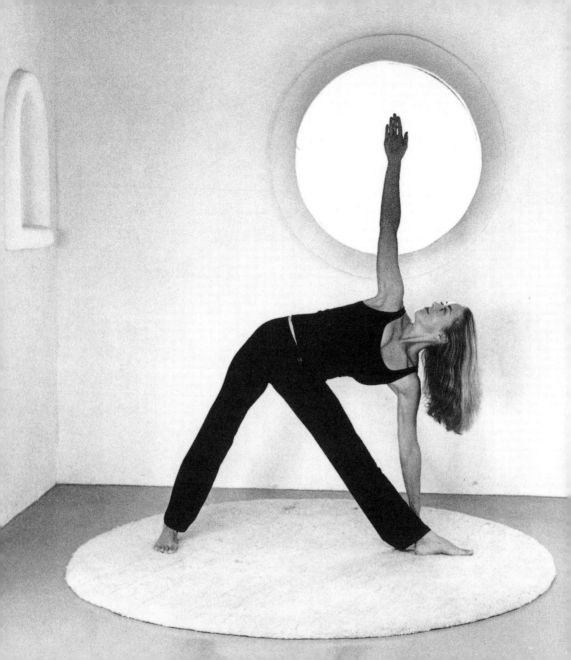

Savasana

To practice *Savasana* is to be awakened to the delicious experience of conscious relaxation. Unlike when we are sleeping, in *Savasana* we are present and proactive as we relax. Through this practice, we develop the ability to relax our body and mind at will, a beneficial tool to have when feeling tired, stressed or overwhelmed.

During *Savasana*, we become aware of any holding on in our body – any muscle tension or spasm – and learn to consciously let go of it. Tension stored in the body for a long time may be difficult to detect at first, and hard to release, but with intention and practice all of the holding on in the body – even of the skin and organs – can be released.

Get in touch with the inner and outer layers of your body and feel them softening. Focus on releasing any holding in of the organs, including the brain. Relax the nerves, the skeleton and all the soft tissues, including the skin, our largest organ. Practice becoming aware of tension stored in the body and just let it go.

The various yoga postures stimulate and activate different energies in the body and nervous system and *Savasana* rebalances these and returns us to a calm and centered space. It is best always to complete a Hatha yoga session with *Savasana* or relaxation.

Extend the duration of your *Savasana* practice if you have been doing a lot of dynamic yoga postures. Generally, 10 to 20 minutes is recommended. With practice you will intuitively tune into your body and know how much time you need to be in *Savasana* to feel relaxed and centered.

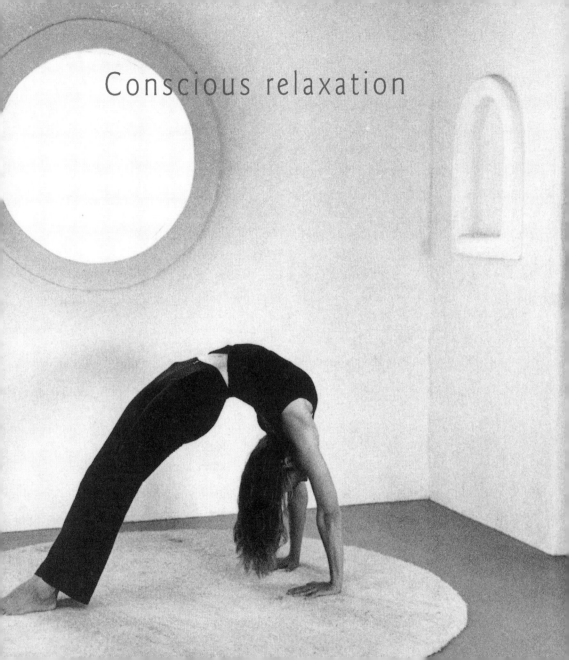

Conscious relaxation

Savasana A

Positioning: Lie flat on your back on the floor with your legs slightly parted, let your feet and legs fall away from each other. Rest your arms on the floor alongside but slightly away from your body, with the palms of your hands facing upward. Tuck your chin in gently and rest the back of your head on the floor. Close your eyes, place an eye bag over your eyes and part your lips slightly to relax your jaw.

Technique: Once in position, resolve not to move or wriggle around. Now's the time to relax completely. Scan your whole body, internally and externally, from superficial muscles to deep tissues, and relax any parts that feel tense. Some common points of holding on are the muscles around the eyes and eyeballs, the jaw and throat, the forehead and neck. Release these completely.

Bring your awareness to a single point of focus. Choose one of the following and return to it whenever you find your mind wandering: the rise and fall of your chest as you breathe; the cool air moving in through your nostrils as you breathe in and the warm air moving out as you exhale; your third eye; or the soft sound of your breathing. A point of focus helps to let go of thinking and empty the mind.

Focus: On relaxing and allowing your breath to flow naturally; do not try to control your breathing. Do not allow yourself to sleep; this is conscious relaxation, an "awake" sleep.

Hold: Remain in this position and state for 10 to 20 minutes after a yoga *asana* practice or whenever you feel the need to relax.

Benefits: This position helps to empty and relax the mind, nervous system and whole body. It helps to restore energy levels, overcome fatigue and release stress.

This **simple** position is highly effective in attaining **complete** relaxation of mind and body. Practice it when you really need to stop and **rest**.

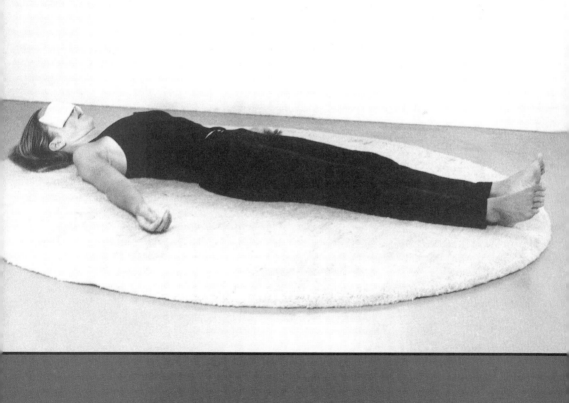

Savasana B

Positioning: Arrange three folded blankets (a single folded blanket, with a stack of two folded blankets on top of it) to make a two-tiered support for your back. Sit on the floor with your legs outstretched at the lower end of the tier. Lie back over the blankets or bolsters, with your lower back resting on the lower half and your upper back on the more raised section. Tuck your chin in and let your feet and legs fall away from each other. Place an eye bag over your eyes.

Technique: Once in position, resolve not to move or wriggle around. Now's the time to relax completely. Scan your whole body, internally and externally, from superficial muscles to deep tissues, and relax any parts that feel tense. Some common points of holding on are the muscles around the eyes and eyeballs, the jaw and throat, the forehead and neck. Release these completely.

Bring your awareness to a point of focus. Choose one of the following and return to it whenever you find your mind wandering: the rise and fall of your chest as you breathe; the cool air moving in through your nostrils as you breathe in and the warm air moving out as you exhale; your third eye; or the soft sound of your breathing.

Focus: On relaxing and allowing your breath to flow naturally; do not try to control your breathing. Do not allow yourself to sleep; this is conscious relaxation, an "awake" sleep.

Hold: Remain in this position and state for 10 to 20 minutes after a yoga *asana* practice or whenever you are feeling blocked in the heart area or are finding it difficult to breathe.

Benefits: This position promotes deep breathing, and opens the heart and lungs. It helps to restore energy levels, overcome fatigue and release stress.

The chest is raised, opening the lungs and allowing deep, full breathing: this is the posture to open hearts!

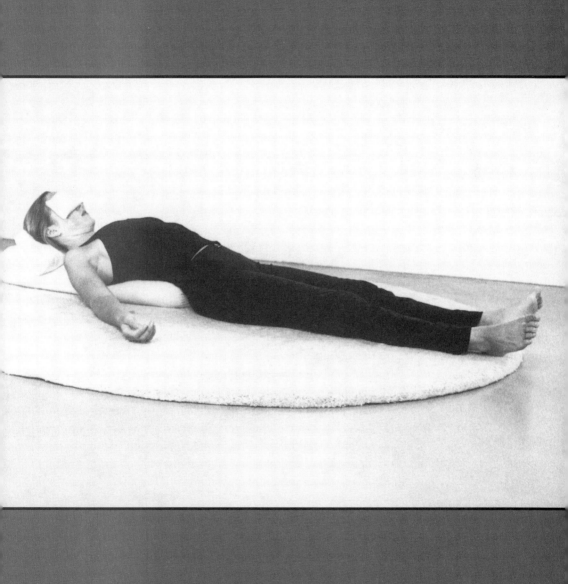

Savasana C

Positioning: Lie flat on the floor on your stomach, with your arms resting by your side. Let your feet and legs relax, and turn your head to rest on one side. Close your eyes and let your mouth open gently.

Technique: Once in position, resolve not to move or wriggle around. Now's the time to relax completely. Scan your body, internally and externally, from superficial muscles to deep tissues, and relax any parts that feel tense. Some common points of holding on are the muscles around the eyes and the eyeballs, the jaw and throat, the forehead and neck. Release these completely.

When you are satisfied that your body is completely relaxed, bring your awareness to a point of focus. Choose one of the following and return to it whenever you find your mind wandering: the cool air moving in through your nostrils as you breathe in and the warm air moving out as you exhale; your third eye; or the soft sound of your breathing. A point of focus helps to let go of thinking and empty the mind.

Focus: On relaxing and allowing your breath to flow naturally; do not try to control your breathing. Do not allow yourself to sleep; this is conscious relaxation, an "awake" sleeping.

Hold: Remain in this position and state for 10 to 20 minutes after a yoga *asana* practice or whenever you feel the need to restore your energy levels.

Benefits: In this position your abdominal organs are massaged. It also helps to empty and relax the mind, nervous system and whole body. It restores energy levels, and helps overcome fatigue and release stress.

A nurturing position where our more **vulnerable** side, the front of the body, is rested and **protected** on the floor.

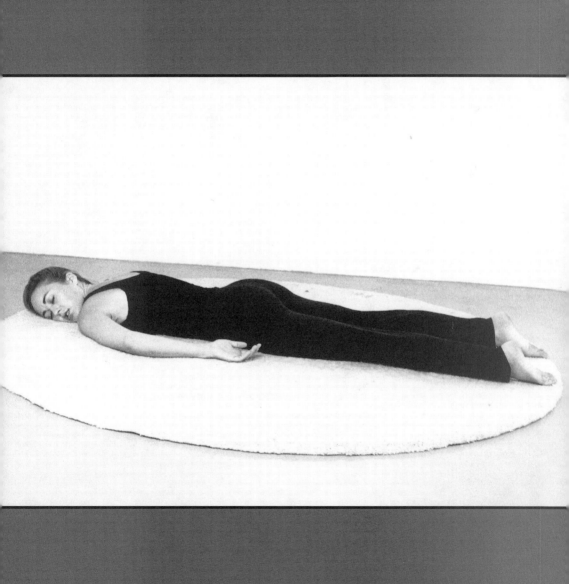

Savasana D

Positioning: Lie flat on the floor on your back with your knees resting over one or more folded blankets or a bolster. Rest your head on a folded blanket and tuck your chin in. With your legs slightly parted, let your feet and legs fall away from each other. Rest your arms on the floor alongside but slightly away from your body. Close your eyes, place an eye bag over your eyes, part your lips slightly, and turn your focus inward.

Technique: Once in position, resolve not to move or wriggle around. Now's the time to relax completely. Scan your body, internally and externally, from superficial muscles to deep tissues, and relax any parts that feel tense. Feel your lower back muscles loosening and relaxing. Some common points of holding on are the muscles around the eyes and eyeballs, the jaw and throat, the forehead and neck. Release these completely.

Bring your awareness to a point of focus. Choose one of the following and return to it whenever you find your mind wandering: the cool air moving in through your nostrils as you breathe in and the warm air moving out as you exhale; your third eye; or the soft sound of your breathing. A point of focus helps to let go of thinking and empty the mind.

Focus: On relaxing and allowing your breath to flow naturally; do not try to control your breathing. Do not allow yourself to sleep; this is conscious relaxation, an "awake" sleeping.

Hold: Remain in this position and state for 10 to 20 minutes after a yoga *asana* practice or whenever your lower back is aching.

Benefits: This position helps to release the lower back muscles. It also helps to empty and relax the mind, nervous system and whole body. It restores energy levels, and helps overcome fatigue, release stress and relieve tired legs.

This **therapeutic** position relieves spasm in the lower back muscles, and **restores** energy to an overworked back, legs and feet.

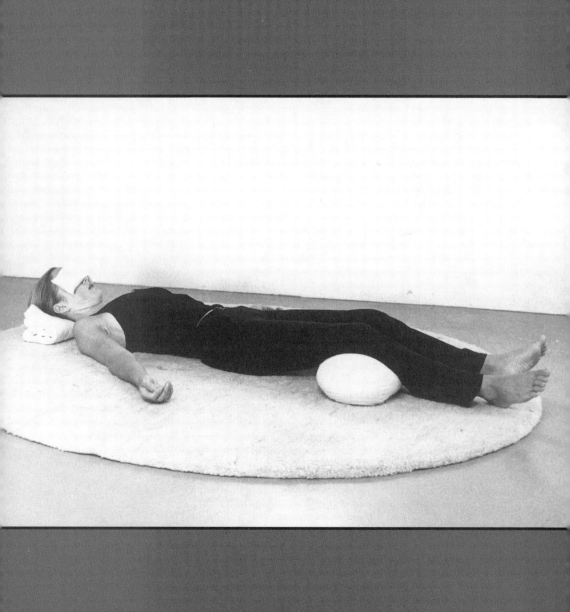

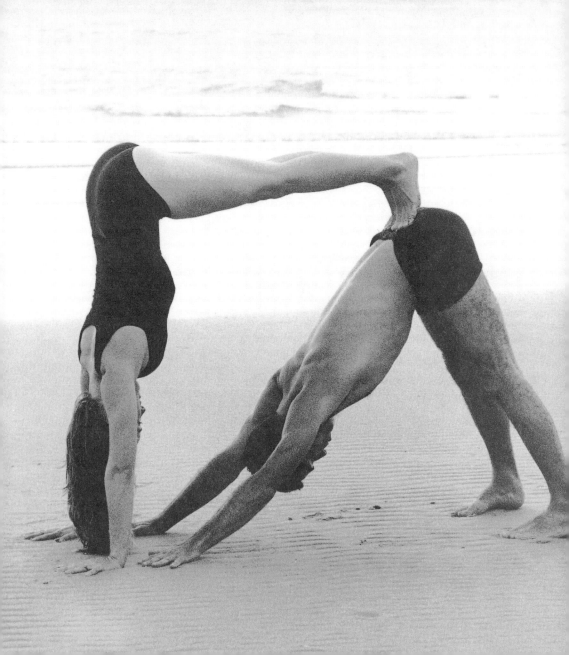

Inverting for health

Give yourself a boost of life with nourishing upside-down poses. We spend most of our lifetime standing, sitting or lying flat, so it makes healthy sense to regularly turn ourselves upside down and reverse the downward pull of gravity on our body.

Because it's the reverse of normal, turning upside down stimulates the cleansing flow of oxygenated blood, which assists in increased nourishment of the body and cell regeneration. Inverting also assists the body to rid itself of illness and disease.

The increased supply of oxygen to the brain, which is a consequence of inverted poses, relieves mental fatigue and promotes clear thinking and good memory. The body's circulatory and other systems are also activated, which can relieve tiredness, cleanse and tone the body, and help to reverse the aging process; aching legs and feet are also relieved.

There are many variations of inverted postures, from simply leaning up against a wall and hanging forward or resting the legs up a wall, to more advanced postures such as the Full Shoulder Stand. Choose one that feels right for you and let your body do the work.

Before attempting the half and full shoulder stand, however, it is recommended that you first learn these postures under the guidance of a yoga teacher.

Don't attempt or practice any inverted poses if you have a sore neck, high blood pressure, a weak heart, brain problems or epilepsy, or during menstruation. If you are pregnant, check with your yoga teacher for some safe variations.

Upside down and healthy

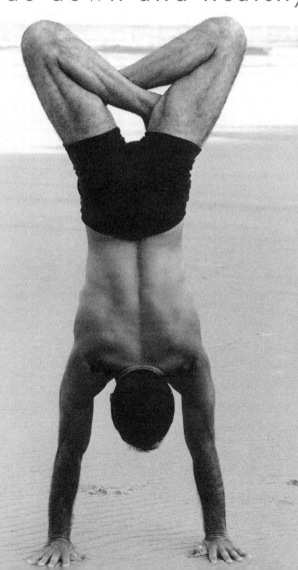

Forward hang (using a wall)

Position: Place your feet hip-width apart about one foot away from a wall and lean back until your buttocks are resting against the wall. As you inhale, move the flesh of your buttocks away from your sitting bones, lift out of your waist and tuck your thumbs into the creases of your elbows and raise them above your head. As you exhale, bend at the hips and hang all the way forward and down, releasing the forehead toward the knees. Tuck your chin in and close your eyes.

Focus: Let your body weight sink to your buttocks and let the wall support you.

Breath: Soft breaths through the nose.

Hold: 10 breaths or 5 to 10 minutes for deep relaxing.

Coming Down: Bend your knees and roll up to a standing position away from the wall.

Benefits: Relieves fatigue, calms the mind and helps overcome stress and anxiety.

When your mind is overworked or your body tired, hang forward and let your worries wash over your back like water.

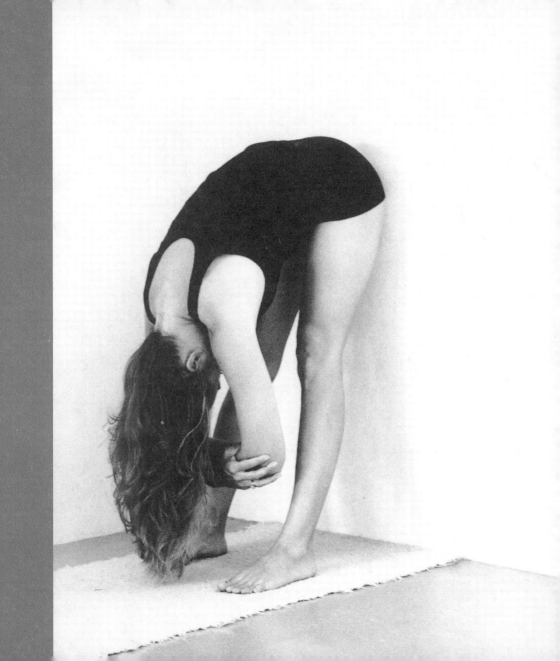

Viparita Karani

VIPARITA – INVERTED: KARANI – PRACTICE

Positioning: Place two or three folded blankets against a wall. Position yourself so that your pelvis is raised on the blankets, and your upper spine, shoulders and head are on the floor. Straighten your legs in an upward position against the wall, bringing your feet together. Your buttocks should be touching the wall. Rest your arms on the floor out to the side, your palms facing upward. Flex your feet so that the soles are parallel to the ceiling and your toes are pointing back to your head. Engage your thigh muscles and push the back of your knees to the wall. Tuck your chin in and relax completely.

Breathing: Breathe evenly through the nose, expanding your chest fully with each inhalation.

Focus: Relax every muscle in your body except for your leg muscles, which remain slightly contracted.

Hold: 10 breaths or 5 to 10 minutes for deep relaxing.

Coming Down: Bend your knees and roll to the side. Rest and come up slowly.

Benefits: This position assists lymphatic drainage and blood flow, and relieves tired, aching feet and legs. It relieves fatigue and helps overcome stress and anxiety.

This posture is simple to practice and deeply relaxing. Inverting your legs in this position restores the body's energy levels. Raising the pelvis cascades energy downward and nourishes the heart.

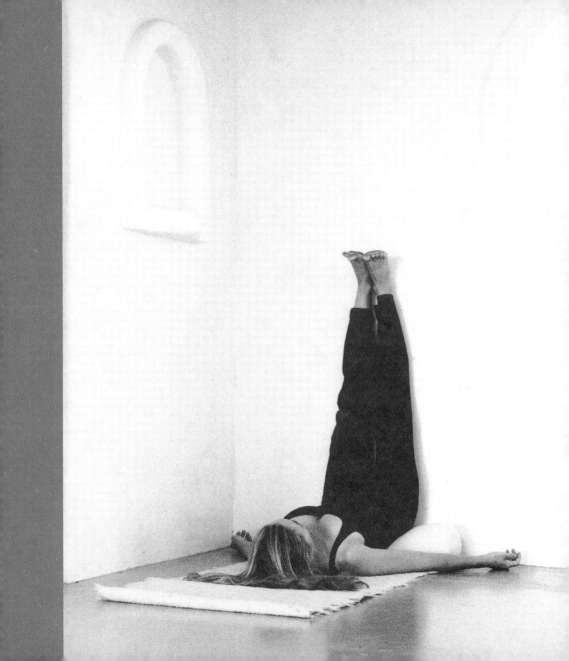

Chair rest

Positioning: Lie flat on your back, resting your arms on the floor with your palms facing upward. Tuck in your chin and close your eyes. Rest your calves along the seat of a chair. There is nothing else to do and nowhere else to go. Relax completely.

Breathing: Breathe evenly through your nose, expanding your chest fully with each inhalation.

Focus: Relax every muscle in your body.

Hold: For 10 breaths or 5 to 10 minutes for deep relaxation.

Coming Down: Bend your knees and roll to the side. Rest and come up slowly.

Benefits: This position assists lymphatic drainage and blood flow, and relieves tired, aching feet and legs. It relieves fatigue and helps overcome stress and anxiety.

Practice this position to **calm**, relax and **restore** yourself after a busy day or whenever you're feeling exhausted. This supported inversion pose has a **nurturing** effect on your whole being. Enjoy!

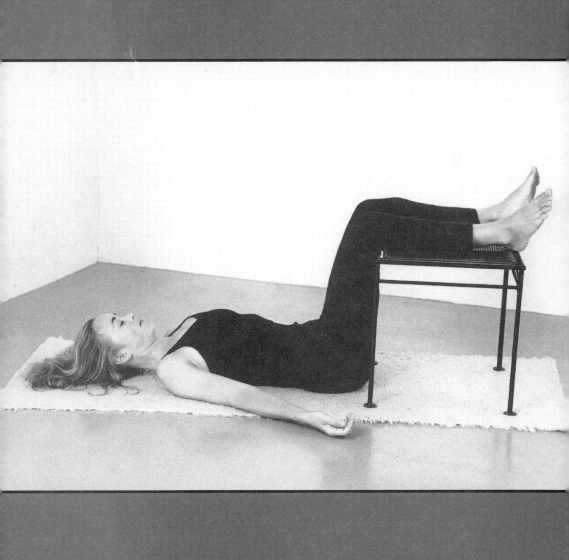

Supported Halasana

HALA – PLOUGH

Positioning: Place two or three folded blankets next to a chair with the folded edges facing inward. Lie with your back over the blankets, your shoulders an inch back from the edge of them and your head on the floor under the chair. Raise your legs and rest the front of your thighs along the seat of the chair. Raise your arms above your head and relax them along the floor.

Breathing: Soft inhalation and exhalation through the nose.

Focus: Relax completely.

Hold: For 10 breaths or 5 to 10 minutes for deep relaxation.

Coming Down: Allow your legs to come down to the floor. Rest, then roll to the side and sit up slowly.

Benefits: This relaxing posture relieves tired feet and legs, calms the nervous system, relieves fatigue, and helps release stress and overcome anxiety.

Precaution: It is recommended that you learn this posture with a yoga teacher before attempting it on your own.

Contraindications: Sore neck, high blood pressure, weak heart, brain problems, epilepsy; pregnancy and menstruation.

This relaxing posture slows your body's physical activity down and allows the brain to relax as the focus is turned inward. When you feel overwhelmed, this posture can be the getaway you need.

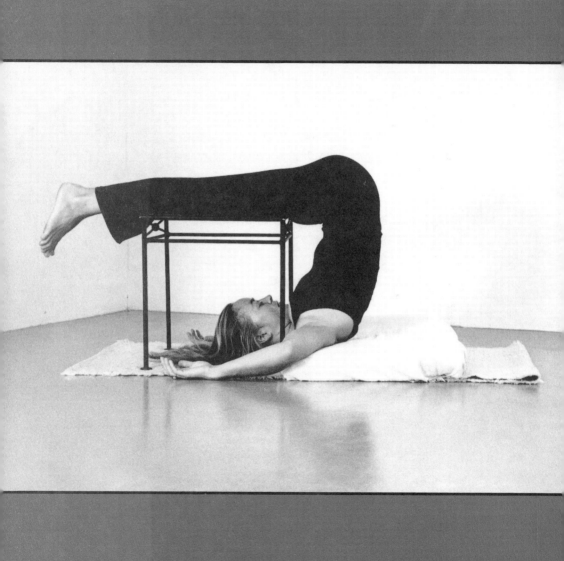

Viparita Karani Mudra

VIPARITA — INVERTED; KARANI — PRACTICE;

MUDRA — CREATING A SEAL

Positioning: Lie on your back on two or three neatly folded blankets, with your shoulders about an inch from the folded edge and with your head on the floor. With your chin tucked in, inhale and bring your legs over your head, place the palms of your hands on your hips for support and straighten your legs halfway, creating a right angle with your torso. Bring your elbows in and support your hips with your hands.

Breathing: Breathe softly through the nose.

Focus: Use a soft eye gaze in the direction of your navel. Keep your shoulders on the blankets. Relax your throat.

Hold: For 10 breaths or as long as comfortable. Release immediately if you feel pressure rising in your head or behind your eyes.

Coming Down: Allow your back and buttocks to drop gently back to the floor. Rest. Slowly roll to one side and sit up when ready.

Benefits: This position strengthens your back and increases blood supply to the whole body. It is especially beneficial in nourishing the glands, and relieves anxiety, headache, fatigue, intestinal and abdominal problems and poor digestion. It helps to improve memory and stimulate the brain, and produces mental calm, peace of mind and all-over vitality.

Precaution: It is recommended that you learn this posture with a yoga teacher before attempting it on your own.

Contraindications: Sore neck, high blood pressure, weak heart, brain problems, epilepsy; pregnancy and menstruation.

This beautiful posture **strengthens** your back while also **cleansing** your whole body. Be in the pose with the breath as your self comes back to life.

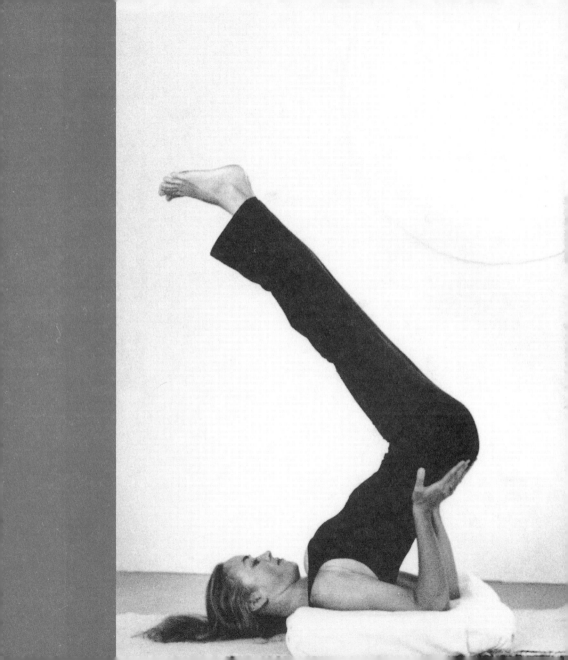

Preparation Sarvangasana

SARVANGA – WHOLE BODY

Positioning: Place two or three folded blankets about one foot out from a wall. Lie on your back with your buttocks on the floor and your legs up the wall. Position the blankets so that the back of your head is on the floor and your shoulders are resting an inch back from the outside edge of the folded blankets. Position your buttocks against the wall. Now, bending your knees, press the soles of your feet against the wall and lift your buttocks, hips and torso up off the floor. Bring your elbows in and support your back with your hands. Straighten your back.

Breathing: Breathe softly through your nose.

Focus: Eye gaze to your navel. Keep your shoulders on the blanket. Relax your throat. Press the soles of your feet against the wall. Keep your back straight. Bring your pubis forward.

Hold: For 10 breaths or as long as comfortable. Release immediately if you feel pressure rising in your head or behind your eyes.

Coming Down: Release your arms, bend your knees and allow your back and buttocks to drop gently back to the floor. Rest.

Benefits: This position allows increased blood supply to the whole body, especially to the glands. It helps to relieve anxiety, headache, fatigue, intestinal and abdominal problems and poor digestion, improves memory, stimulates the brain, and improves all-over vitality.

Precaution: It is recommended that you learn this posture with a yoga teacher before attempting it on your own.

Contraindications: Sore neck, high blood pressure, weak heart, brain problems, epilepsy; pregnancy and menstruation.

Inverting the body restores energy levels, helps to reverse the aging process, and refreshes the mind and outlook on life. This posture uses the support of a wall, allowing you to perform the posture easily.

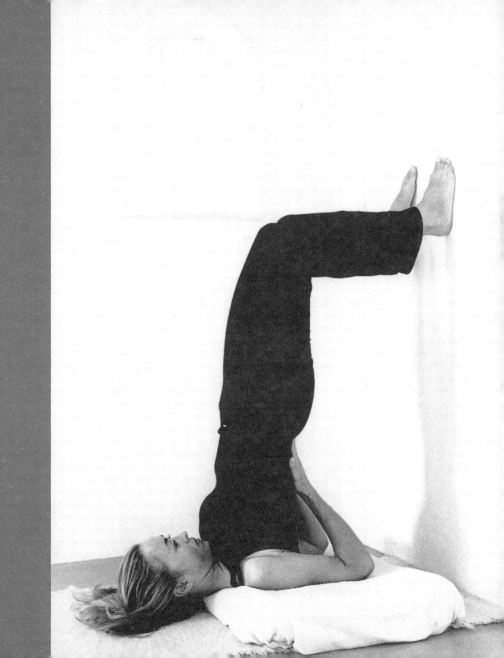

Salamba Sarvangasana

Positioning: Lie back on two or three neatly folded blankets, with your shoulders about an inch from the blanket's folded edge and your head on the floor. Bend your knees and bring your feet up against your buttocks. Raise your legs off the floor, placing the palms of your hands onto your upper back for support. Slowly move your legs into a vertical position, forming a straight line. Your elbows should be shoulder-width apart and, along with your shoulders, support and lift your body.

Breathing: Breathe softly and evenly through your nose.

Focus: Eye gaze directed to the navel. Relax your throat, neck, head and facial muscles. Keep your body straight.

Hold: For 10 breaths or as long as comfortable. Release immediately if you feel the pressure rising in your head or behind your eyes.

Coming Down: Exhale as you gently allow your legs, back and buttocks to return to the floor. Remove the blankets and rest your body flat on the floor.

Benefits: This position allows increased blood supply to the whole body, especially the glands. It helps to relieve anxiety, headache, fatigue, intestinal and abdominal problems and poor digestion, stimulates the brain, and improves memory and all-over vitality.

Precaution: It is recommended that you learn this posture with a yoga teacher before attempting it on your own.

Contraindications: Sore neck, high blood pressure, weak heart, brain problems, epilepsy; pregnancy and menstruation.

The shoulder stand is one of the most superior of yoga *asanas*. Known as the queen of postures, it maintains a healthy mind and body, and assists in preventing illness and disease.

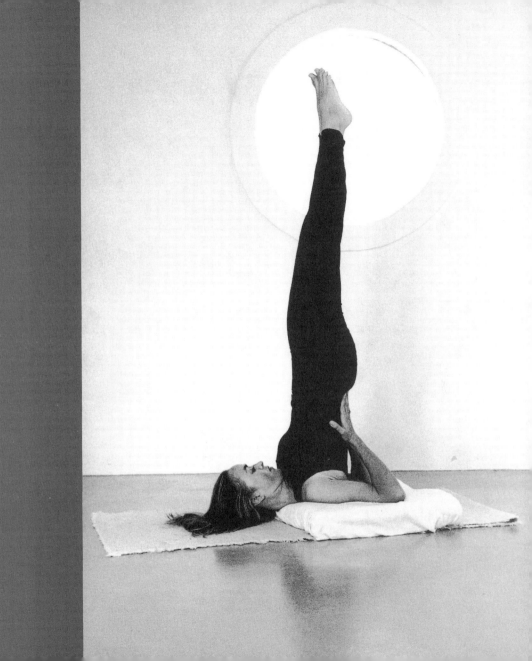

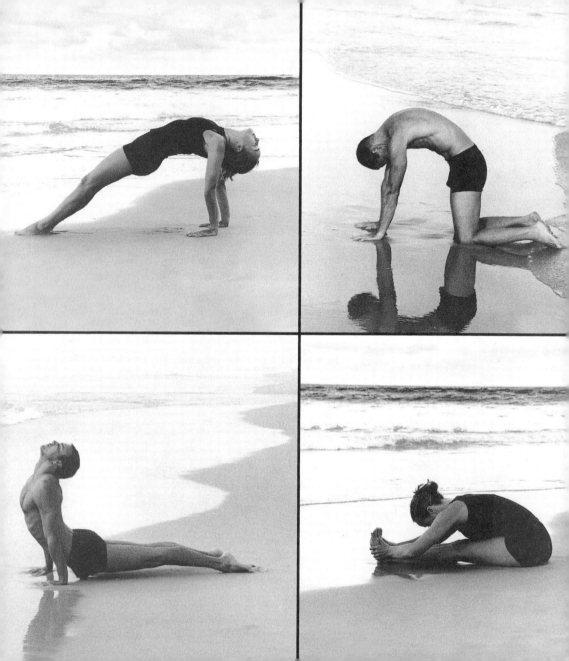

General sequences

Surya Namaskar A

SURYA – SUN: NAMASKAR – SALUTE

Technique: Breathing through your nose, move in and out of the postures with the breath. Keep your body moving to create a rhythmic, flowing sequence.

A dynamic sequence, traditionally practiced before sunrise to greet the new day. Body and breath flow energetically to create intense heat and to stimulate circulation. Practice this sequence to warm up, cleanse, tone and refresh mind and body.

POSITION I *NAMASTE*

Close your eyes and hold your hands in prayer position in front of your heart to center yourself in stillness. Get in touch with your breathing and your heart center.

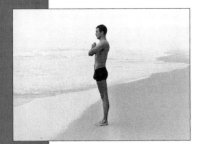

POSITION 2 *TADASANA*

Stand with your feet together, arms by your side. Focus forward at eye level and get in touch with your whole body from your feet up. Straighten your spine and center your bodyweight around it.

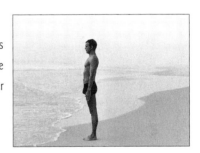

POSITION 3 *URDHVA HASTASANA*

INHALE and raise your arms above your head, bringing your palms together, and look up to your hands. Extend your body upward from your hips, feeling your whole body elongating.

POSITION 4 *UTTANASANA*

EXHALE and release your arms out to the sides. Bend forward at the hips, bring your palms to the floor, and forehead and torso in toward your knees. Straighten your legs (if you have lower back pain, you should keep your knees bent), tuck your chin in and direct your focus up toward your navel.

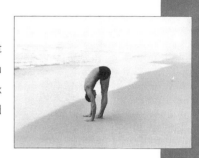

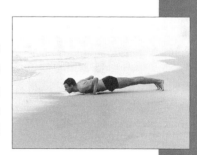

POSITION 5 *UTTANASANA* LOOKING UP

INHALE and place your hands on the floor beside your feet. Looking up, extend and lengthen your spine.

POSITION 6 *CATURANGA DANDASANA*

EXHALE and step or lightly jump your feet back, straighten your legs and arms into a straight line, keeping your body raised off the floor, then slowly release your body down to the floor, keeping your elbows in close to your body. If you have the strength, keep your whole body slightly off the floor; if not, rest your legs and chest to the floor but keep your leg muscles activated.

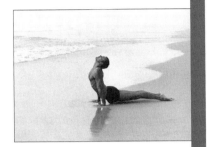

POSITION 7 *URDHVA MUKHA SVANASANA*

INHALE and roll onto the tops of your feet, lifting your pelvis and bringing your chest up and forward, straightening your arms. Roll your shoulders back and open up your chest. Extend your legs away and squeeze your buttocks, extending out from your lower back. Either look forward or close your mouth and drop your head back, looking beyond your forehead.

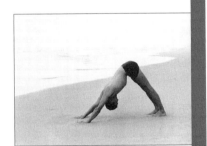

POSITION 8 *ADHO MUKHA SVANASANA*

EXHALE and lift your buttocks and hips. Roll your feet so that your heels go back to the floor. Spread your fingers wide apart and extend up through your arms. Relax your head and chest and look at a point between your feet on the floor. Contract your thigh muscles upward and extend your hips, pubis and buttocks upward without lifting your heels. Elongate your spine. Rest here for five deep, full breaths.

POSITION 9 *UTTANASANA* LOOKING UP

INHALE and lightly step or jump your feet to your hands, looking forward as in Position 5.

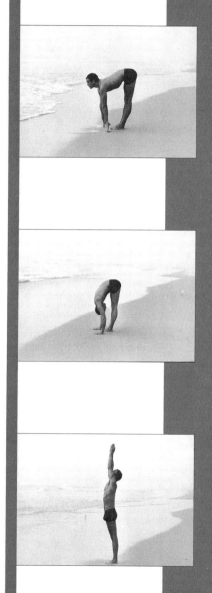

POSITION 10 *UTTANASANA*

EXHALE and bring your head into your knees as in Position 4.

POSITION 11 *URDHVA HASTASANA*

INHALE, extend your arms straight out to the sides and come up to standing position. Stretch your arms above your head, bring your palms together, and look up as in Position 3.

EXHALE and release your arms to your sides and return your eye focus to a point in front as in Position 2.

Practice this sequence a few times to warm up and stretch the whole body.

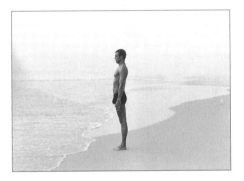

Surya Namaskar B

SURYA – SUN; NAMASKAR – SALUTE

Technique: Breathing through your nose, move in and out of each posture with each inhalation and exhalation to create a rhythmic and dynamically flowing sequence.

Combining stretching and strengthening postures,

Surya Namaskar B synchronizes the movement of the

body with the breath to create intense internal heat. Empty

your mind and go with the flow.

POSITION 1 *NAMASTE*

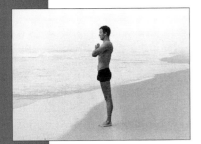

Close your eyes and hold your hands in prayer position in front of your heart to center yourself in stillness. Get in touch with your breathing and your heart center.

POSITION 2 *TADASANA*

Stand with your feet together, arms by your side. Focus forward at eye level and get in touch with your whole body from your feet up. Straighten your spine and center your bodyweight around it.

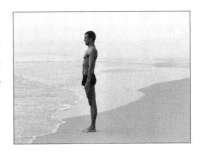

POSITION 3 *UKTASANA*

INHALE and bend your knees, swinging your arms behind you and then forward in prayer position to above your head. Look up to your hands, tuck your buttocks under, and extend out from the waist halfway up, keeping your knees bent.

POSITION 4 *UTTANASANA*

EXHALE and, keeping your palms together, bring your arms down as you bend forward at the hips, then bring your palms to the floor and forehead and torso in toward the knees. Straighten your legs (if you have lower back pain, you should keep your knees bent), tuck your chin in and direct your focus up toward your navel.

POSITION 5 *UTTANASANA* LOOKING UP

INHALE and cup your fingers on the floor in front of your feet. Looking up, extend and lengthen your spine, concaving your lower back.

POSITION 6 *CATURANGA DANDASANA*

EXHALE and step or lightly jump the feet back into the plank position, then slowly release your body down to the floor, keeping your elbows in close to your body, the legs locked and facing down. If you have the strength, keep your whole body slightly off the floor; if not, rest your legs and chest to the floor but keep your leg muscles activated.

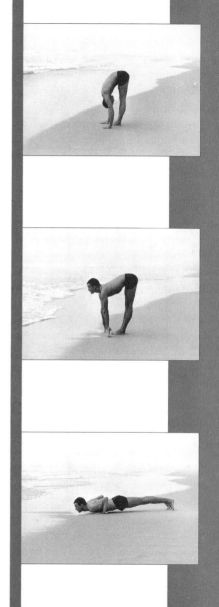

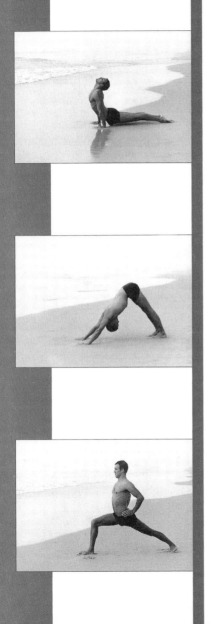

POSITION 7 *URDHVA MUKHA SVANASANA*

INHALE and roll onto the tops of your feet, lifting your pelvis and bringing your chest up and forward, straightening your arms. Roll your shoulders back and open up your chest. Extend your legs away and squeeze your buttocks, extending out from your lower back. Either look forward or drop your head back, looking beyond your forehead and keeping your mouth closed.

POSITION 8 *ADHO MUKHA SVANASANA*

EXHALE and lift your buttocks and hips. Roll your feet so that your heels go back to the floor.

POSITION 9 *VIRABHADRASANA I –*
RIGHT FOOT FORWARD

INHALE and turn your left foot out 45 degrees. Step the right foot forward about one yard. Place your hands on your hips and bend your right leg to create a 90-degree angle. Stretching out from your hips, rotate the left hip forward to align it with the right hip. Keep the back leg muscles activated. Roll your shoulders back and look forward.

POSITION 10 *CATURANGA DANDASANA*

EXHALE and step your right foot back. Straighten your legs and come down, keeping your body raised off the floor and your elbows in toward the body.

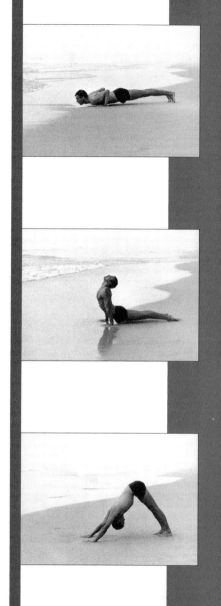

POSITION 11 *URDHVA MUKHA SVANASANA*

INHALE and roll onto the tops of your feet, bringing the front of your body up through your shoulders and straightening your arms, as in Position 7.

POSITION 12 *ADHO MUKHA SVANASANA*

EXHALE and lift your buttocks and hips. Roll your feet so that your heels go back to the floor, as in Position 8.

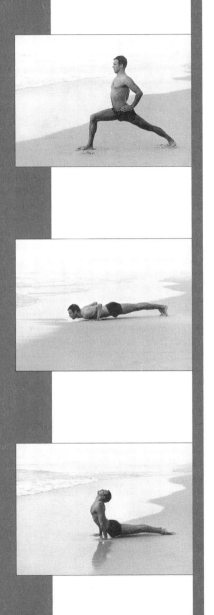

POSITION 13 *VIRABHADRASANA I –*
LEFT FOOT FORWARD

INHALE and turn your right foot out 45 degrees. Step your left foot forward about one yard. Place your hands on your hips and bend your left leg to create a 90-degree angle. Stretching out from your hips, rotate the right hip forward to align it with the left hip. Keep both legs activated and the back leg straight. Roll your shoulders back and look forward.

POSITION 14 *CATURANGA DANDASANA*

EXHALE and step your left foot back. Straighten your legs and come down, keeping your body raised off the floor and your elbows in toward the body.

POSITION 15 *URDHVA MUKHA SVANASANA*

INHALE and roll onto the tops of your feet, bringing the front of your body up through the shoulders and straightening your arms, as in Position 7.

POSITION 16 *ADHO MUKHA SVANASANA*

EXHALE and lift your buttocks and hips. Roll your feet so that your heels go back to the floor. Spread your fingers wide apart and extend up through your arms. Relax your head and look at a point between your feet on the floor. Contract your thigh muscles upward and lift your hips, pubis and buttocks without lifting your heels. Elongate your spine. Rest here for 5 deep, full breaths.

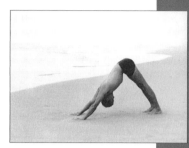

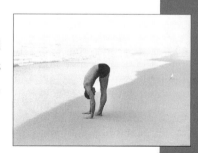

POSITION 17 *UTTANASANA* LOOKING UP

INHALE and step or lightly jump your feet to your hands. Place your hands on the floor in front of your feet and look up. Extend and lengthen your spine, concaving your back.

POSITION 18 *UTTANASANA*

EXHALE and bring your palms to the floor beside your feet and your forehead and torso in toward your knees. Straighten your legs (if you have lower back pain, you should keep your knees bent), tuck your chin in and direct your focus toward your navel.

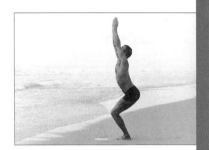

POSITION 19 *UKTASANA*

INHALE and bend your knees, swinging your arms behind you and then forward in prayer position to above your head. Look up to your hands, tuck your buttocks under, and extend out from the waist halfway up, keeping your knees bent.

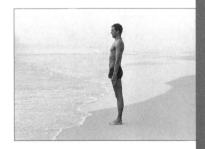

POSITION 20 *TADASANA*

EXHALE and straighten your body, releasing your arms to your sides and standing with your feet together, focusing forward.

Practice this sequence a few times to warm up and stretch the whole body.

Surya Namaskar C

SURYA – SUN: NAMASKAR – SALUTE

Technique: Breathing through your nose, move in to each of the postures on inhalation and out of each posture on exhalation. Keep your body moving to create a rhythmic, flowing sequence.

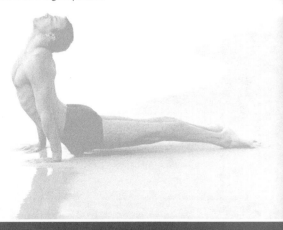

This third Salute to the Sun sequence develops

strength and willpower. Practice it to stretch

and tone the whole body.

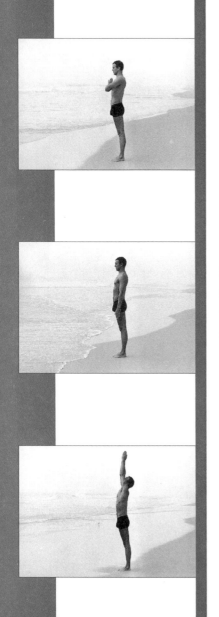

POSITION 1 *NAMASTE*

Close your eyes and hold your hands in prayer position in front of your heart to center yourself in stillness. Get in touch with your breathing and heart center.

POSITION 2 *TADASANA*

Stand with your feet together, arms by your side. Focus forward at eye level and get in touch with your whole body from your feet up. Straighten your spine and center your bodyweight around it.

POSITION 3 *URDHVA HASTASANA*

INHALE and raise your arms above your head, bringing your palms together, and look up to your hands. Extend your body upward from your hips, feeling your whole body elongating.

POSITION 4 *UTTANASANA*

EXHALE and release your arms out to the sides. Bend forward at the hips, bring your palms to the floor and forehead and torso in toward your knees. Straighten your legs (if you have lower back pain, you should keep your knees bent), tuck your chin in and direct your focus up toward your navel.

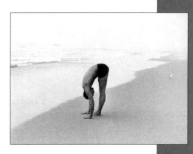

POSITION 5 *UTTANASANA* LOOKING UP

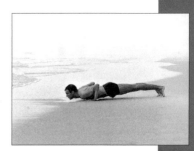

INHALE and cup your fingers on the floor in front of your feet. Looking up, extend and lengthen your spine, concaving your back.

POSITION 6 *CATURANGA DANDASANA*

EXHALE and step or lightly jump the feet back into the plank position, then slowly release your body down to the floor, keeping your elbows in close to your body, the legs locked and facing down. If you have the strength, keep your whole body slightly off the floor; if not, rest your legs and chest to the floor but keep your leg muscles activated.

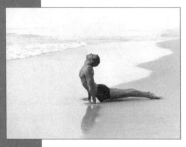

POSITION 7 *URDHVA MUKHA SVANASANA*

INHALE and roll onto the tops of your feet, lifting your pelvis and bringing your chest up and forward, straightening your arms. Roll your shoulders back and open up your chest. Extend your legs away and squeeze your buttocks, extending out from your lower back. Either look forward or drop your head back, looking beyond your forehead.

POSITION 8 *ADHO MUKHA SVANASANA*

EXHALE and lift your buttocks and hips. Roll your feet so that your heels go back to the floor.

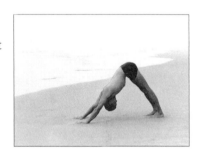

POSITION 9 *UKTASANA*

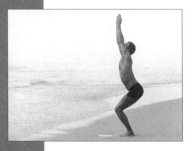

INHALE and lightly step or jump your feet to your hands. Looking forward, bend your knees and swing your arms behind you then forward, bringing your hands into prayer position above your head. Tuck your buttocks under and extend out from the waist halfway up, keeping your knees bent and looking up or straight ahead. Hold this position for 5 full breaths.

EXHALE and straighten your body, releasing your arms to your sides and standing with your feet together, focusing forward.

Practice this sequence a few times to warm up and stretch the whole body.

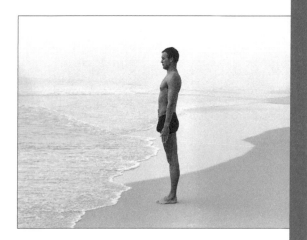

East-west sequence

Technique: Breathing through your nose, move in and out of each posture with deep, full breathing to create a rhythmic flow.

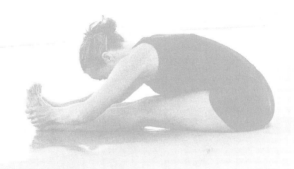

Moving from *Purvottanasana* (*purva* – east) to *Pascimottanasana* (*pascima* – west), this is a dynamic flow between the two opposites: prone and supine, back and front, introverted and extroverted, east and west.

Practice to invigorate yourself!

POSITION 1 *DANDASANA*

Sit with your back straight, legs outstretched and arms straight with palms to the floor beside your hips, fingers facing forward. INHALE.

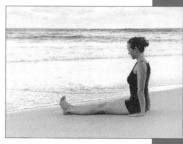

POSITION 2 *PASCIMOTTANASANA*

EXHALE as you bend at the hips to extend forward over your legs with your arms outstretched.

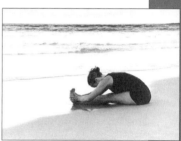

POSITION 3 *PURVOTTANASANA*

INHALE as you come up. Place your hands on the floor behind your hips with your fingers facing forward. Press your feet to the floor as you lift your hips, torso and legs high off the floor and drop your head back. Lock your arms and legs as you extend your toes to the floor and lift from your abdominal and pubic muscles. Bring your eye focus to the tip of your nose.

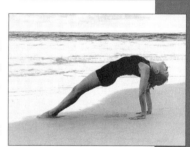

EXHALE as you release your legs and buttocks to the floor and extend your body forward all the way over your legs, as in Position 2.

Keep moving between these positions with the in and out breaths for 10 cycles. To release, lie flat on the floor and rest with your knees drawn into your chest.

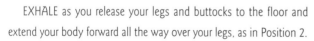

is gentle spinal

loosens

spine,

reasing the

culation to

body's

tems. Practice

se curls as a

rm-up for the

ole body

to assist in

eding up your

tabolism.

Cat curls

POSITION I

Kneel with your hands shoulder-width apart on the floor, your knees hip-width apart.

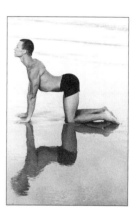

POSITION 2

INHALE and look up to the tip of your nose, making your back concave.

POSITION 3

EXHALE, tucking your chin under into the neck, and stretch your entire back upward – like a stretching cat.

Repeat this cycle 10 times slowly, inhaling up and exhaling under, focusing on smooth, even breaths through your nose.

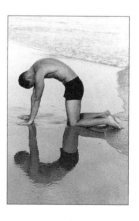

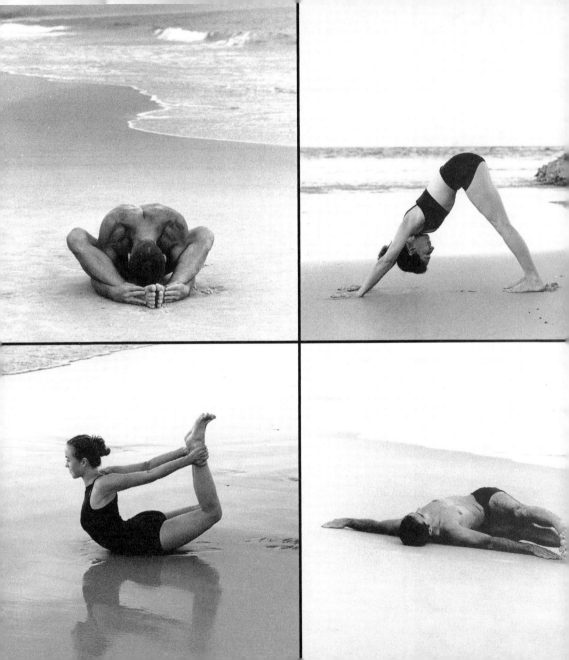

Remedial sequences

Ways to remedy health problems naturally, such as through yoga practice, are also a means to getting to know and understand – as well as heal – thyself. However, because natural therapies don't always offer the fastest relief and require self-participation and effort, people often opt for quick-fix conventional treatments.

Taking the steps to heal thyself naturally has other, ongoing benefits. In the process of understanding a health problem, you develop an awareness of the physical, mental, emotional and spiritual connection at work within. When you become more tuned in to your body you're more likely to detect ill health in its early stages.

General ailments often just require some focused attention, gentle stretching and breath work to release tension and holding in sore areas. This approach can often help prevent the onset of more severe symptoms. Yoga helps prevent disease and illness naturally with postures that cleanse the organs, activate the glands, restore the body's various systems and exercise the respiratory muscles, as well as releasing stress and tension from the whole body.

Give your body the chance to breathe, release and relax naturally with these healing postures. Use common sense: avoid practicing any postures that don't feel right, and if your condition is severe, consult a qualified and experienced remedial yoga teacher or medical practitioner before attempting them.

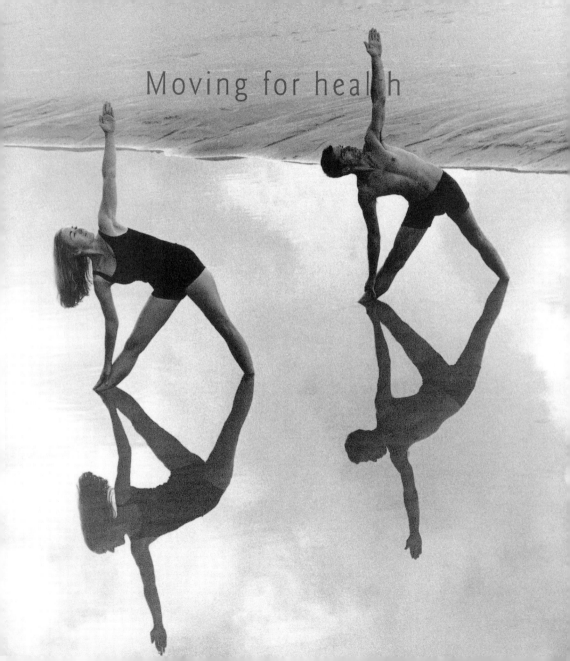

Moving for health

Computer tension

Headaches, sore neck and shoulders, chest tightness and aching eyes are just a few of the more common complaints experienced by computer operators. Simple but regular stretching and frequent breaks greatly reduce tension and help to maintain a sense of vitality throughout the working day. Discipline is required at first, but once in the swing of it, your body will automatically "remember" this healthy habit. Take regular breaks and slip into this routine to save your body, mind and eyes.

Begin with Meditation (Chapter 3), Cat curls (Chapter 6) and East-west sequence (Chapter 6).

When working at a computer, we often forget to **breathe** fully. Turn your power box on with **frequent**, deep, full breathing and stretching exercises for good health and energy levels.

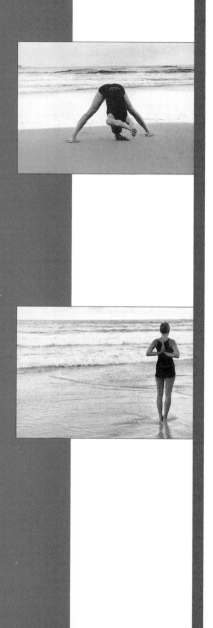

1. *PADOTTANASANA* III – FOOT-LEG EXTENSION POSE

Stand with your feet about five feet apart. Interlock your fingers behind you. Inhale and raise your arms, extending up and out from your waist. Exhale and bend at your hips, slowly bringing your arms over your head and your hands toward the ground. Lock your legs, lean forward into the balls of your feet and feel the opening in the backs of your legs. Release your spine, head and neck toward the floor, keeping your shoulders lifted. Eye focus to the navel. Hold for 5 to 10 even breaths through the nose. Inhale to come up.

2. *NAMASTE* BEHIND THE BACK

While standing or sitting, reach behind your back and bring your hands into the *Namaste*, or prayer position. Feel your shoulders and chest opening up and allow any tension and stiffness in your hands to release. Hold for 10 breaths. Practice this posture frequently while working at the computer to release tension and promote correct breathing.

3. SIDE SHOULDER STRETCH

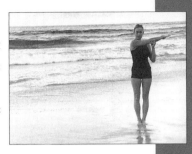

Standing, raise your right arm and, using your left hand to support it, rest your arm across the front of your body, stretching the shoulder and upper arm.

After a few breaths, repeat with your other arm. Practice frequently to loosen tight muscles.

4. *DHANURASANA* – BOW POSE

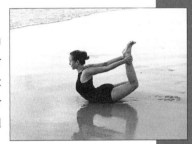

Lie on your stomach, bend your knees, lifting your feet behind you in the air, and press your pubis to the floor. Inhale and bring your hands back to hold your ankles while raising your head and chest off the ground. Draw your knees in toward each other, open your shoulders and lift your chest. Lightly squeeze the buttocks. Hold for 5 full breaths. Exhale to release down. Rest and repeat twice.

5. SHOULDER STRETCH

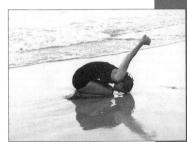

Sit with your buttocks on your heels, forehead to the floor and fingers interlocked behind your back. Inhale, and then on the exhale, raise your arms and release them over your head, moving your hands toward the floor. Breathe for 5 to 10 breaths.

Complete with Forward hang (Chapter 5), Deep, full breathing (Chapter 2) and *Savasana* B (Chapter 4).

you practice

s sequence,

go of

inking and

ax. Allow your

dy to rest and

mply

eathe. There is

thing to do

d nowhere

go.

Fatigue

Overcome tiredness and fatigue with gentle postures that increase circulation and restore the body's energy levels. Fatigue can be caused by working too much, thinking too much, stress, anxiety, a poor diet and bad sleeping patterns. Bring yourself back to life with this nurturing sequence and remember to practice deep, full breathing to oxygenate your brain.

Begin with Deep, full breathing (Chapter 2), Cat curls (Chapter 6) and Forward hang (Chapter 5).

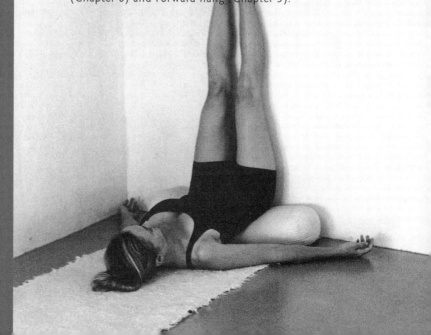

1. VIPARITA KARANI

Place a bolster or some folded blankets next to a wall. Lie with your legs up the wall, your hips and pelvis elevated on a bolster so that they are higher than your heart. Relax your upper back, shoulders, neck and head on the floor, and rest your arms on the floor to your sides or above your head to open the chest and allow deep, full breathing. Rest in this gentle, relaxed, inverted position for 5 to 10 minutes.

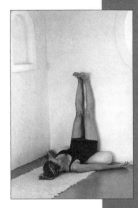

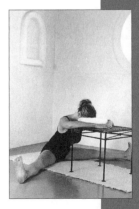

2. FORWARD REST

Kneel on the floor. Bring your big toes together and move your knees apart. Sit back between the heels and on the soles of your feet. Inhale and walk your hands forward along the floor, lengthening your spine, and rest your forehead on the floor. Keep your buttocks on your heels and keep your arms extended forward to create a two-way stretch along the spine. Hold for 10 breaths. Inhale to release.

3. KONASANA WITH HEAD RESTING ON A CHAIR

Sit with your legs wide apart facing a chair. Rest your forehead on a folded blanket on the seat of the chair. Rest your arms on the chair and breathe fully. Relax in this pose for a few minutes.

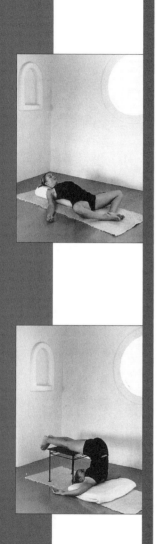

4. *SUPTA BADDHA KONASANA* LYING OVER A BOLSTER
LENGTHWISE – SUPINE BOUND ANGLE POSE

Sit with outstretched legs, a bolster or folded blankets extending lengthwise behind you. With your buttocks on the floor and your lower back touching the end of the bolster, exhale and lie back over the bolster, resting your head and upper back on it. Tuck in your chin and extend your arms to the sides. Bring the soles of your feet together and release your hips as your knees drop to the floor. Focus on breathing fully and opening out your chest, lungs and heart. Rest in this position for 5 to 10 minutes.

5. SUPPORTED *HALASANA* – PLOUGH POSE

Place two or three folded blankets next to a chair with the folded edges facing inward. Lie with your back over the blankets, your shoulders on the edge of them and your head on the floor under the chair. Raise your legs up and over to rest the thighs along the seat of the chair. Relax your arms above your head on the floor. Hold for 5 to 10 minutes. To release, slowly raise your legs from the chair and return them slowly to the floor, resting on your upper back and shoulders.

Complete this sequence with Preparation *Salamba Sarvangasana* (Chapter 5), Meditation (Chapter 3) and *Savasana* D (Chapter 4).

RSI

Repetitive strain and pressure on the fingers and wrists can cause tightening of the joints and muscles and inhibit circulation. By softening your shoulder and neck muscles, where stress and tension are often stored, you can help to prevent and relieve painful and limiting repetitive strain and carpal tunnel conditions. This therapeutic sequence promotes circulation in the arms and releases upper body tightness.

Do not practice postures where your arms bear your bodyweight, as this can cause a flare-up of the condition.

Begin with Meditation (Chapter 3), Deep, full breathing (Chapter 2) and Forward hang (Chapter 5).

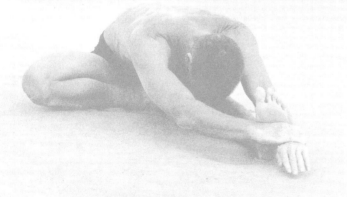

Be mindful in each pose by breathing and **releasing** into your hands and arms. Visualize the **flow** of cleansing and **healing** oxygenated blood through your limbs.

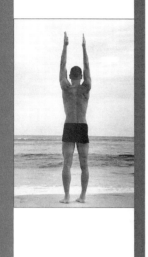

1. URDHVA HASTASANA – RAISED HAND POSE

Stand with the arms by your sides, your feet hip-width apart and your eyes focusing forward. Inhale and raise your arms above your head, keeping your hands shoulder-width apart. Relax the shoulders down. Extend upward from the waist, through the torso and arms. Hold for 10 breaths, release, rest and repeat.

2. SALABHASANA – LOCUST POSE

Lie on your stomach and place your arms alongside your body, your palms facing upward. Rest your forehead on the floor. Inhale to raise your head, chest, arms, shoulders and legs off the floor, activating and strengthening your entire back; only the front of your torso and hips should be in contact with the floor. Focus forward and hold the position for 10 even breaths. Inhale to release down. Rest and repeat.

3. FORWARD *SUKHASANA*

Sit in an easy cross-legged position. Fold your arms behind your back, bringing your thumbs into the crease of the opposite elbow. Inhale, lifting out from the waist. Exhale to extend and release forward and down. Rest your forehead on the floor or a bolster. Hold for 10 full breaths. Inhale to release up.

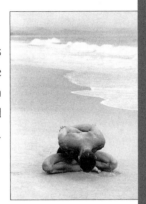

4. *KURMASANA* VARIATION –
TORTOISE POSE

Sitting with the soles of your feet together, place your hands under your knees and slide your feet forward. Let your torso and head come down, and bring your hands around to meet your feet. Hang forward, relaxing your head, shoulders and spine. Hold the position for 10 full breaths. Inhale slowly to come up.

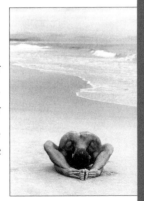

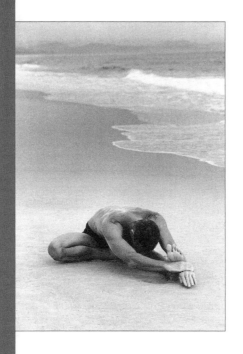

5. *JANU SIRSASANA* – HEAD TO KNEE POSE

Sit with your legs outstretched and bend your right leg up, placing the heel close to your groin, with the sole of your foot facing upward. Release the right knee down to the floor, opening up your right hip. Inhale and lift the front of your body. Exhale and extend forward and down to lie your torso over the length of your left leg, elongating the hamstrings and softening your back muscles. Breathe softly and fully for 5 breaths. Inhale, come up out of the posture, and repeat on the other side.

Headache

When you feel the onset of a headache, these postures will increase the flow of oxygenated blood to your head and brain, and release tension and strain. Focus on breathing out waste products with each exhalation, and taking in new life with each inhalation.

Begin with Meditation (Chapter 3), Alternate-nostril breathing (Chapter 2) and Forward hang (Chapter 5).

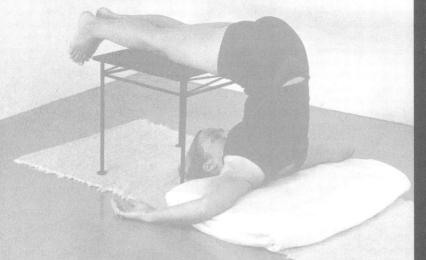

Detoxify and **purify** your mind and body with these postures that **soothe** the nervous system, increase circulation and **release** waste products stored in the body.

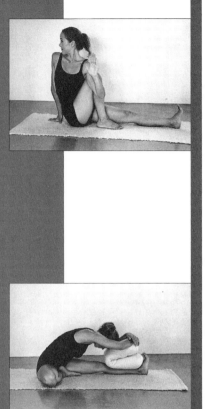

1. MARICYASANA TWIST – INDIAN SAGE POSE

Sit with your legs outstretched and bend your right leg, placing your foot on the floor near your groin so that your thigh is touching your abdomen. Place your right hand on the floor behind your right hip. Lock your left arm in front of your right knee. Inhale and lift up from your hips, thinning your waist. Exhale and twist to look over your right shoulder. Keep your left leg muscles activated. Release into the twist for 5 breaths. Release, come back to center, and repeat on the other side.

2. JANU SIRSASANA – HEAD TO KNEE POSE

Sit with your legs outstretched and bend your right leg up, placing the heel close to your groin, with the sole of your foot facing upward. Release the right knee down to the floor, opening up your right hip. Inhale and lift the front of your body. Exhale and extend forward and down to lie your torso over the length of your left leg, resting your head on a pillow, elongating the hamstrings and softening your back muscles. Breathe softly and fully for 5 breaths. Inhale, come up out of the posture, and repeat on the other side.

3. SUPPORTED *HALASANA* – PLOUGH POSE

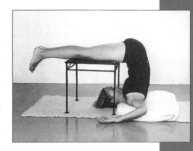

Place two or three folded blankets next to a chair with the folded edges facing inward. Lie with your back over the blankets, your shoulders on the edge of them and your head on the floor under the chair. Raise your legs up and over to rest the thighs along the seat of the chair. Relax your arms above your head on the floor. Hold for 5 to 10 minutes. To release, slowly raise your legs from the chair and return them slowly to the floor, resting on your upper back and shoulders.

4. *SUPTA BADDHA KONASANA* LYING OVER A BOLSTER LENGTHWISE – SUPINE BOUND ANGLE POSE

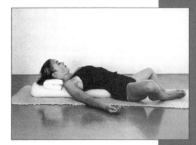

Sit with outstretched legs, a bolster or folded blankets extending lengthwise behind you. With your buttocks on the floor and your lower back touching the end of the bolster, exhale and lie back over the bolster, resting your head and upper back on it. Tuck in your chin and extend your arms to the sides. Bend your knees and bring the soles of your feet together, allowing your legs to splay open and releasing your hips as your knees drop to the floor. Focus on breathing fully and opening out your chest, lungs and heart. Rest in this position for 5 to 10 minutes.

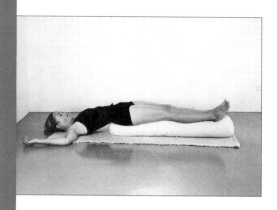

5. *SETU BANDHA* – SUPPORTED BRIDGE POSE

Rest your legs, buttocks and lower back over a long bolster or rolled blankets positioned lengthwise. Rest your head, shoulders and upper back on the floor, and allow your arms to relax on the floor above your head. This slight inversion position rests the heart, calms the mind and soothes the nervous system, helping relieve tension and headache. Rest in this pose for 10 minutes. To release out of the position, bend your knees and roll to one side.

Complete this sequence with Cat curls (Chapter 6), Deep, full breathing (Chapter 2) and *Savasana* B (Chapter 4).

Anxiety and stress

When you're stressed or anxious, find the time to stop, relax and enter a quiet place within. This simple sequence of postures offers the space to unwind and clear your head, incorporating twisting and back-strengthening postures to cleanse and prepare for change. Practice each posture with the breath and release into a new perspective on life so that even overwhelming problems may become more manageable.

Begin with Cat curls (Chapter 6), *Surya Namaskar* A (Chapter 6) and Forward hang (Chapter 5).

In times of hardship and worry, **nurture** yourself with postures that take you away from all your cares and **immerse** you in calm.

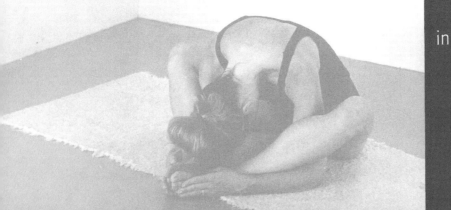

1. *KURMASANA* VARIATION – TORTOISE POSE

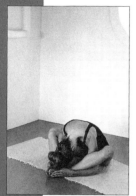

Sitting with the soles of your feet together, place your hands under your knees and slide your feet forward. Let your torso and head come down, and bring your hands around to meet your feet. Hang forward, relaxing your head, shoulders and spine. Hold the position for 10 full breaths. Inhale slowly to come up.

2. *BHARADVAJASANA* – INDIAN SAGE POSE

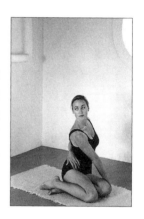

Sit on your buttocks and place your feet next to your right hip. Put your left foot beneath your right foot. Inhale up out of your waist and twist right. Place your right hand by your left knee and your left hand on the floor behind your left hip. Inhale, wrap your left arm around your back and hold your right hip. Looking right, rotate your left shoulder back. Hold for 5 breaths, release and change sides.

3. *NAVASANA* – BOAT POSE

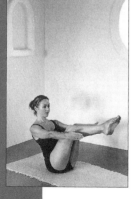

Sit on the floor and find your balance forward on your sitting bones. Bend and raise your legs halfway in toward your chest, and extend your arms out parallel to your lower legs. Move around until you feel centered. Lift your lower back in and up so that your spine isn't collapsing. Hold for 5 to 10 breaths, release, rest and repeat twice. If you have the strength, aim to straighten your legs.

4. *SETU BANDHA* – SUPPORTED BRIDGE POSE

Rest your legs, buttocks and lower back over bolsters or rolled blankets positioned lengthwise. Rest your head, shoulders and upper back on the floor, and allow your arms to relax on the floor above your head. This slight inversion position rests the heart, calms the mind and soothes the nervous system, helping relieve tension and headache. Close your eyes and rest in this pose for 10 minutes. To release out of the position, bend your knees and roll to one side.

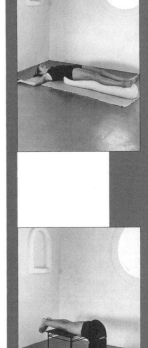

5. SUPPORTED *HALASANA* – PLOUGH POSE

Place two or three folded blankets next to a chair with the folded edges facing inward. Lie with your back over the blankets, your shoulders on the edge of them and your head on the floor under the chair. Raise your legs up and over to rest the thighs along the seat of the chair. Relax your arms above your head on the floor. Hold for 5 to 10 minutes. To release, slowly raise your legs from the chair and return them slowly to the floor, resting on your upper back and shoulders.

Complete this sequence with *Viparita Karani* (Chapter 5), Meditation (Chapter 3) and *Savasana* B (Chapter 4).

ve your veins a

st and let the

od flow

sily with

side-down

stures that

eanse and

store vibrant

alth to your

gs.

Varicose veins and tired legs

Lack of movement, standing for long periods or muscle constriction can cause poor circulation through the legs, possibly leading to weakening of the veins, soreness and even blood clots. Promote blood flow, release waste products and relieve fatigue with these gentle inverted positions. Practice them as often as possible to help prevent the onset of varicose veins and restore energy levels.

Begin with Meditation (Chapter 3), *Surya Namaskar* B (Chapter 6) and East-west sequence (Chapter 6).

1. LEGS UP THE WALL A

Lie flat on your back with your legs up against a wall. Press your buttocks firmly into the wall and press your lower back down to the floor. Rest your arms out to the side with your palms facing upward. Tuck your chin in slightly, close your eyes and hold for 25 deep, full breaths. Proceed to Legs up the wall B.

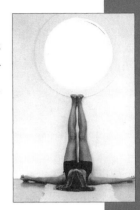

2. LEGS UP THE WALL B

Lie flat on your back with your legs up against a wall. Press your buttocks firmly into the wall and press your lower back down to the floor. Slide your legs apart to a comfortable position where you feel a gentle opening in the inner leg muscles and groin. Extend your arms out to the sides and rest the back of your hands on the floor. Tuck your chin in slightly, close your eyes and hold for 25 deep, full breaths. To release out of this position, bring your knees to your chest, roll to one side and come up slowly.

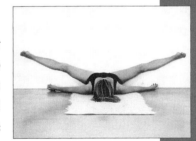

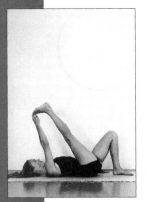

3. *SUPTA PADANGHUSTASANA* –
LYING DOWN STRETCH LEG POSE

Lie on your back, bend your left leg, and place the left foot on the floor toward your left hip. Inhale and raise your right leg, holding onto your foot with your right hand. Soften the hamstring and hip areas with each exhalation breath, releasing the leg down. Hold for 5 to 10 breaths. Inhale to release and repeat on the other side. Hold on to a belt around your foot if you can't reach it with your hand.

4. *SETU BANDHA* – SUPPORTED
BRIDGE POSE

Lie on your back over bolsters or rolled blankets positioned lengthwise. Rest your head, upper back and shoulders on the floor, and your arms above your head. This position rests the heart and soothes the nervous system, and relieves tension and headache. Rest for 10 minutes. To release out of the position, bend your knees and roll to one side.

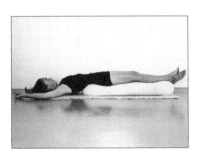

5. CHAIR REST

Lie on your back, arms by your sides and chin tucked in. Rest your calves along the seat of a chair. Close your eyes and focus on your soft breathing. Hold for 5 to 10 minutes. Release by lifting your legs off the chair and resting on your right side.

Complete the sequence with Supported *Salamba Sarvang-asana* (Chapter 5), Meditation (Chapter 3) and *Savasana* D (Chapter 4).

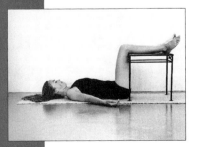

Poor digestion

Poor digestion can be a by-product of stress and "holding on" physically and emotionally. Stimulate digestion with these postures that tone the digestive and abdominal organs, massage and release tension in the stomach muscles and activate the intestines. Complement this sequence with abdominal massage, walking and lots of deep, full breathing.

Begin with Deep, full breathing (Chapter 2), *Surya Namaskar* A (Chapter 6) and *Surya Namaskar* B (Chapter 6).

Get your digestive system **moving** with these postures that twist and deeply **massage** your internal organs.

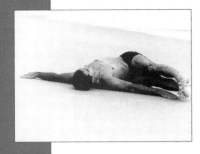

1. JATHARA PARIVARTANASANA – STOMACH TURN POSE

Lie on your back with your arms extended out to the sides, palms facing downward. Exhale and raise your legs to create a 90-degree angle to your torso. Keeping your back flat on the floor and your head centered, lock your legs, lift your hips slightly to the left and slowly release your legs down to the right. If possible, hover your feet beside your right hand without touching the floor, otherwise let your legs rest on the floor. Hold for 5 breaths, then inhale your legs up to center and repeat on the other side. Repeat the full sequence twice.

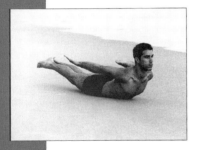

2. SALABHASANA – LOCUST POSE

Lie on your stomach and place your arms alongside your body, your palms facing upward. Rest your forehead on the floor. Inhale to raise your head, chest, arms, shoulders and legs off the floor, activating and strengthening your entire back; only the front of your torso and hips should be in contact with the floor. Focus forward and hold the position for 10 even breaths. Inhale to release down. Rest and repeat.

3. *PARIVRTTA PARSVAKONASANA* VARIATION – REVOLVED SIDEWAYS ANGLE POSE

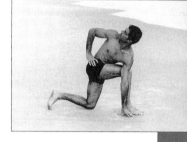

From a standing position with your hands on your hips, step your right foot forward about five feet and, squaring your hips to the front, lunge the right leg forward into a right angle. Rest your left knee on the floor. Inhale and raise your left arm. Exhale and turn to look over your right shoulder while placing your left hand on the floor beside your right foot. Working with the breath, inhale to lift out from your waist, then exhale to twist further to the right. Hold for 5 breaths. Inhale to release out of the pose and change sides.

4. *MARICYASANA* TWIST – INDIAN SAGE POSE

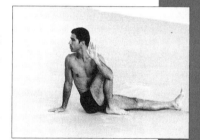

Sit with your legs outstretched and bend your right leg, placing your foot on the floor near your groin so that your thigh is touching your abdomen. Place your right hand on the floor behind your right hip. Lock your left arm in front of your right knee, pressing your knee into your arm. Inhale and lift up from your hips, thinning your waist. Exhale and twist to look over your right shoulder. Keep your left leg straight in front and the muscles activated. Hold the position – and release into the twist for 5 breaths. Release, come back to center, and repeat on the other side.

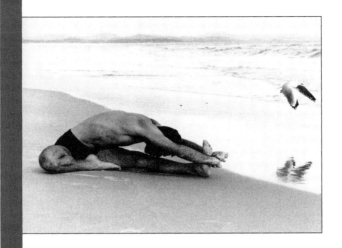

5. JANU SIRSASANA – HEAD TO KNEE POSE

Sit with your legs outstretched and bend your right leg up, placing the heel close to your groin, with the sole of your foot facing upward. Release the right knee down to the floor, opening up your right hip. Inhale and lift the front of your body. Exhale and extend forward and down to lie your torso over the length of your left leg, elongating the hamstrings and softening your back muscles. Breathe softly and fully for 5 breaths. Inhale, come up out of the posture, and repeat on the other side.

Complete the sequence with *Salamba Sarvagasana* (Chapter 5), Deep, full breathing (Chapter 2) and *Savasana* C (Chapter 4).

Poor circulation

Poor circulation can result in chill pains, cold extremities and lack of body heat. Activate your inner fire with dynamic twisting, standing and upside-down poses. Begin this sequence with *Surya Namaskar* A, B or C (Chapter 6), where the body and breath flow dynamically to create intense heat and stimulate circulation throughout the body.

When you're feeling sluggish, you can use this sequence to increase the flow of **oxygenated** blood throughout your body and **regenerate** your body and mind.

1. *UTTANASANA* – EXTENSION POSE

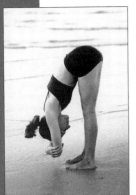

Stand with your feet hip-width apart and interlock your thumbs into your elbows. Exhale to bend at the hips and release your upper body forward and down. Tuck your chin in and focus up to your navel. While breathing deeply and fully, relax your head, neck and shoulders, release your spine and stretch the backs of your legs. Hold for 10 breaths, then bend your knees, inhale and come up slowly.

2. *ADHO MUKHA SVANASANA* – DOWN FACE DOG POSE

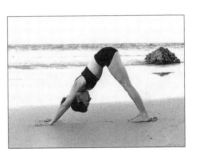

Kneel on the floor, extend your arms forward and step your feet back. Tucking your toes under, lift your buttocks and straighten your legs. Release your heels to the floor. Soften your chest through your shoulders. Gaze softly in the direction of your feet. Hold for 5 to 10 breaths. Exhale as you release down, then rest.

3. *URDHVA MUKHA SVANASANA* – UP FACE DOG POSE

Lie on your stomach with your arms bent and the palms of your hands on the floor beside your shoulders. Inhale and raise your head, torso and legs off the floor. Roll your shoulders back to open up your chest. Keep your legs and arms locked. Focus forward or gently drop your head back. Hold for 10 breaths, expanding the chest fully. Exhale to release down and rest.

4. ARDHA MATSYENDRASANA VARIATION – HALF FISH LORD POSE

Sit with your legs extended out straight. Bend your left leg, placing the foot under the right leg and on the outside of the right buttock. Bend your right leg and place the right foot on the outside of your bent left knee. Place your left arm over your right knee. Inhale and turn to look over your right shoulder, placing your right hand behind you on the ground for support. Working in the pose, inhale to lift out from the waist, and exhale to release deeper into the twist. After 5 full breaths, exhale to release and repeat on the opposite side.

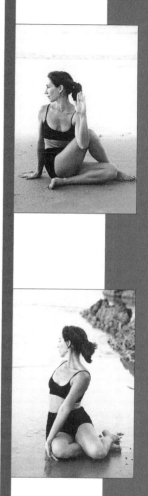

5. BHARADVAJASANA – INDIAN SAGE POSE

Sit on your buttocks and bend your legs sideways to sit next to your left hip. Place your right foot beneath your left foot. Inhale up out of your waist and twist your head and torso to the right. Place your left hand beside your right knee and your right hand around your back to hold on to your left hip. Looking over your right shoulder, rotate your right shoulder and elbow back. Hold for 5 breaths, then release and change sides.

Complete the sequence with *Salamba Sarvangasana* (Chapter 5), Alternate-nostril breathing (Chapter 2) and *Savasana* D (Chapter 4).

elp **shed** weight

om a sluggish

ody with these

ostures that aim to

timulate

etabolism.

Over-weightness

Over-weightness can be caused by an underactive thyroid gland — the gland that regulates growth hormones and the metabolism. Practice this sequence to speed up your metabolic rate.

Begin the sequence with *Suyra Namaskar* A, B or C to warm up and activate the body's internal cleansing process.

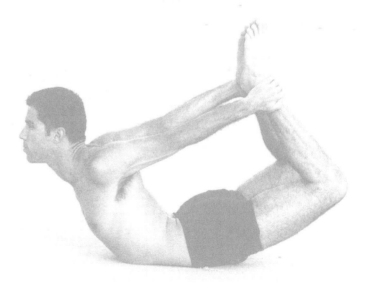

1. NAVASANA – BOAT POSE

Sit on the floor and find your balance on your sitting bones. Move around until you feel centered. Bend and raise your legs halfway in toward your chest, and extend your arms out parallel to your lower legs. Lift your lower back in and up so that your spine isn't collapsing. Hold for 5 to 10 breaths, release, rest and repeat twice. If you have the strength, aim to straighten your legs.

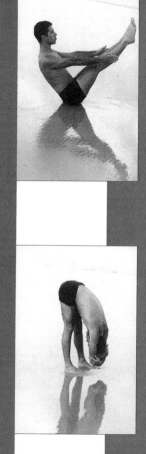

2. UTTANASANA – EXTENSION POSE

Stand with your feet hip-width apart and interlock your thumbs into the crease of the opposite elbow. Inhale to raise your arms above your head. Exhale to bend at the hips and release your arms and upper body forward and down. Tuck your chin in and focus toward your navel. While breathing deeply and fully, relax your head, neck and shoulders, release your spine and stretch the backs of your legs. Hold for 10 breaths, then bend your knees, inhale and come up slowly.

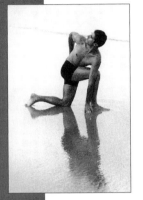

3. PARIVRTTA PARSVAKONASAN VARIATION – REVOLVED SIDEWAYS ANGLE POSE

From a standing position, step your right foot forward about five feet and, squaring your hips to the front, lunge the right leg forward into a right angle. Rest your left knee on the floor. Exhale and turn to look over your right shoulder while placing your left hand on the floor beside your right foot. Rest your right hand on your right hip. Working with the breath, inhale to lift out from your waist, exhale, and twist to the right. Hold for 5 breaths. Inhale and change sides.

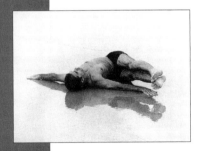

4. JATHARA PARIVARTANASANA – STOMACH TURN POSE

Lie on your back with your arms extended out to the sides, palms facing down. Exhale and raise your legs to create a 90-degree angle to your torso. Keeping your back flat on the floor and your head centered, lock your legs, lift your hips slightly to the left and slowly release your legs down to the right. Hover your feet beside your right hand. Hold for 5 breaths, then inhale your legs up to center and repeat on the other side. Repeat the full sequence twice.

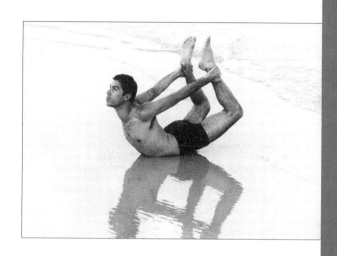

5. DHANURASANA – BOW POSE

Lie on your stomach, bend your knees, lifting your feet behind you in the air, and press your pubis to the floor. Inhale and bring your hands back to hold your ankles while raising your head and chest off the ground. Focus on drawing your head upward, your knees together, opening up your shoulders and lifting your chest. Look forward and lightly squeeze the buttocks. Hold for 5 full breaths. Exhale to release down, rest and repeat twice.

Complete the sequence with Cat curls (Chapter 6), *Viparita Karani* (Chapter 5) and *Savasana* B (Chapter 4).

oid the pain of

iatica by

aintaining

orrect

osture. Ideally,

oid chairs

together and get

to the habit of

tting on the

oor to keep your

ps and legs open

nd energized.

Sciatica

Give relief to nerve compression and pain through the hips, buttocks and legs with postures to open up constricted areas and promote healthy circulation. Stretch deeply and consciously in this sequence, allowing your breath to release your muscles and soothe your nervous system.

Begin with Meditation (Chapter 3), Cat curls (Chapter 6) and Forward hang (Chapter 5).

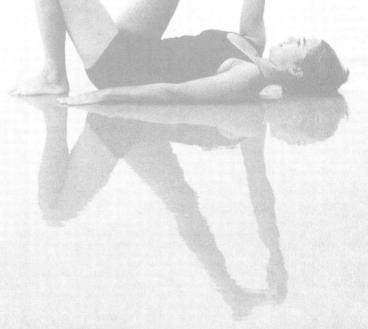

1. SIDE LEG RAISE

Lie on your left side with your legs outstretched. Rest on your left elbow and support your head with your left hand. Inhale and raise your right leg. If you can, hold onto the big toe with the first two fingers of your right hand. If not, hold onto your leg wherever you can reach. Stay in the posture for 5 to 10 breaths. With each exhalation, draw the leg closer toward your head, getting in touch with the release in the inner leg and pelvic muscles.

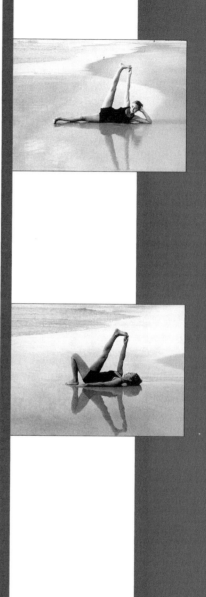

2. SUPTA PADANGHUSTASANA – LYING DOWN LEG STRETCH POSE

Lie on your back, bend your left leg, and place the left foot on the floor toward your left buttock. Inhale and raise your right leg, holding onto your foot with your right hand. Hold onto a belt wrapped around the right foot if you can't reach your foot. Moving with the breath, release into the stretch in the hamstring and hip areas by softening with each exhalation and allowing the leg to gently release forward and down. Hold for 5 to 10 breaths. Inhale to release and repeat on the other side.

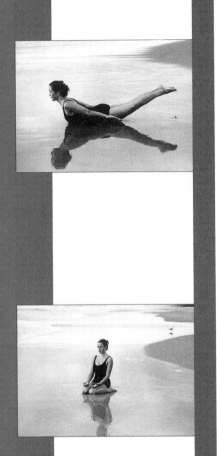

3. *SALABHASANA* – LOCUST POSE

Lie on your stomach and place your arms alongside your body, your palms facing upward. Rest your forehead on the floor. Inhale to raise your head, chest, shoulders, arms and legs off the floor, activating and strengthening your entire back; only the front of your torso and hips should be in contact with the floor. Focus forward and hold the position for 10 even breaths. Inhale to release down, rest and repeat.

4. *VIRASANA* – HERO POSE

Sit with your buttocks on your ankles, then slide your heels out to the sides so your buttocks release to the ground and you are sitting between your heels. At this point, decide whether you will need to sit on some blankets to relieve any tightness in your legs, knees or ankles. Draw your knees in toward each other. Stretch the sides of your torso upward. Roll back your shoulders and open your chest. Rest the backs of your hands on your knees. Breathe for 5 to 10 breaths.

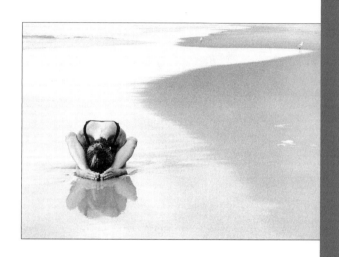

5. *KURMASANA* VARIATION – TORTOISE POSE

Sitting with the soles of your feet together, place your hands under your knees and slide your feet forward. Let your torso and head come down, and bring your hands around to meet your feet. Hang forward, relaxing your head, shoulders and spine. Hold the position for 10 full breaths, releasing into the buttocks and hips. Inhale slowly to come up.

Complete the sequence with Preparation *Salamba Sarvangasana* (Chapter 5), Deep, full breathing (Chapter 2) and *Savasana* A (Chapter 4).

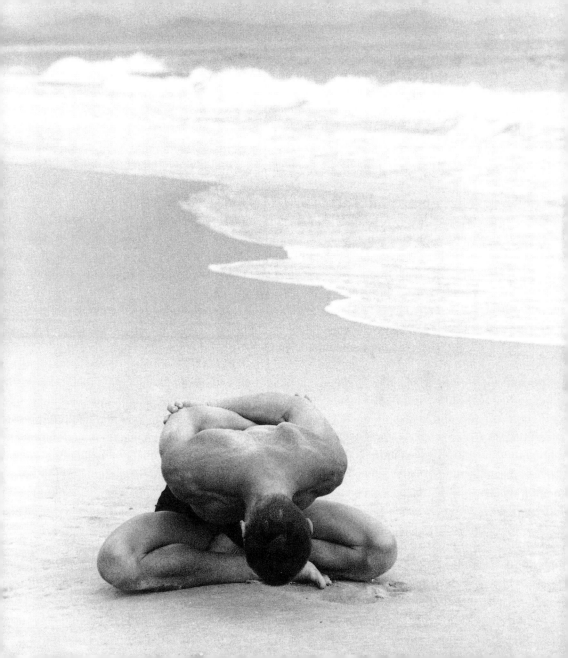

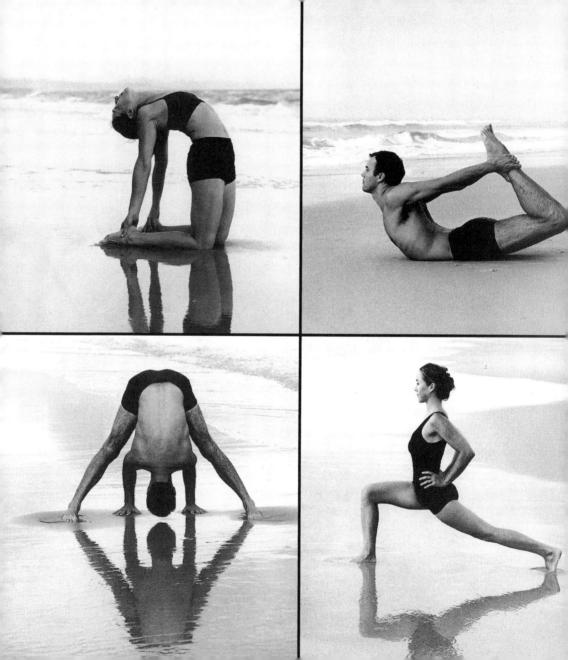

Sport focus

Whether outdoor or indoor activities, sports are healthy for the body and mind.

Like yoga, sports develop mental and physical focus, strength, grace and endurance. In striving to perform better at a sport, we refine our movements, positioning and timing, developing our skill and focus. Likewise when practicing yoga regularly, our postures improve and we experience greater physical ease, skill and fluidity. The experience of being one with a sport and one with a yoga posture is similar.

However, some sports can cause physical problems if played repetitively, and we can develop incorrect breathing patterns that lead to stress, tension and physical discomfort. Specific yoga postures for particular sports can counterbalance repetitive positions and prevent muscle tightness by preparing the body for the activity – warming up – and strengthening weak points.

Add flexibility to your game with these specific sports sequences designed to release tight areas, balance and realign your body, help develop mental focus and concentration, as well as improve lung capacity, breathing and endurance levels.

Take a deep breath and find the point of balance between sharpness and calmness, strength and flexibility, to give your game a natural edge.

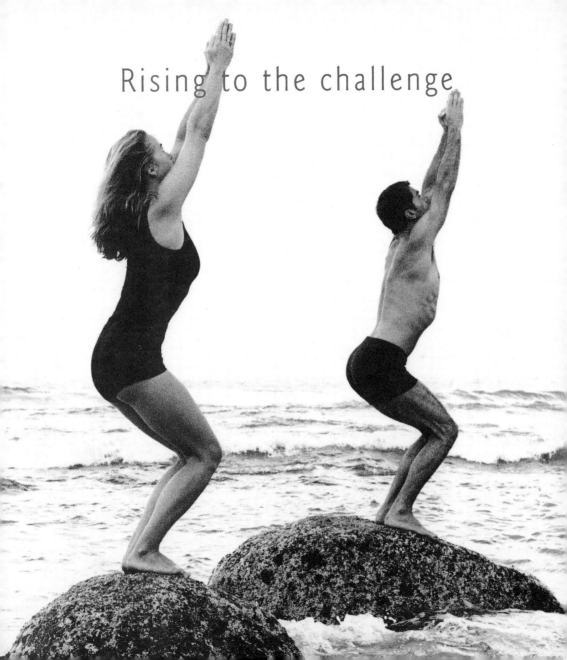

Rising to the challenge

Running, jogging and walking

Running, jogging or walking is like meditation: "time out" to clear the head as well as tone muscles, burn excess body fat and increase circulation and lung capacity. Before you take off, practice this sequence to strengthen your lower back and stretch your leg muscles. Once on track, practice maintaining smooth, even breathing, even when moving fast. Breathe evenly, allowing your body to warm up with the breath. Stay on soft dirt or sand to engage more muscles in the feet and legs and to avoid jarring the joints on hard surfaces. Focus on keeping your posture upright, your back loose, and distributing your bodyweight evenly.

Begin with Alternate-nostril breathing (Chapter 2), *Surya Namaskar* A (Chapter 6) and *Surya Namaskar* C (Chapter 6).

Make each movement a **mindful** experience. Get in touch with your body and be fully **present** in every step you take.

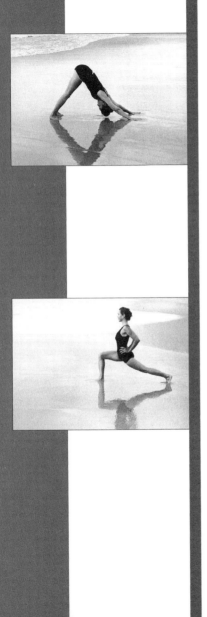

1. ADHO MUKHA SVANASANA –

DOWN FACE DOG POSE

Kneel on the floor, extend your arms forward and step your feet back. Tucking your toes under, lift your buttocks and straighten your legs. Release your heels to the floor, hip-width apart. Soften your chest through your shoulders. Have a soft eye gaze in the direction of your feet. Hold for 5 to 10 breaths. Exhale as you release down, then rest.

2. LEG LUNGE

Begin from a kneeling position, place your hands on your hips and step your right foot forward. Inhale and lift out from your waist. Exhale and lift your left knee and leg off the ground. Keeping your right knee bent and your thigh at a 90-degree angle, drop your left knee down toward the floor to create a stretch in the left quadriceps and the front of the hip. Lift up and down slowly for 5 breaths, releasing further with each exhalation. Inhale to come out of the position, return to kneeling and repeat on the left side.

3. PASCIMOTTANASANA – FORWARD BEND POSE

Sit on the floor with your legs extended out straight and activated. Lift the fleshy part of your buttocks, roll onto your sitting bones and tilt your pelvis forward. Use a belt around your feet and keep your back upright if you can't rest forward. Inhale to lift and extend your pubis, stomach and chest. Exhale to release down and lie over your outstretched legs. Keep both legs locked and the toes working back toward your head. Direct your eye focus toward your feet. Hold for 5 to 10 deep, full breaths. Inhale to release.

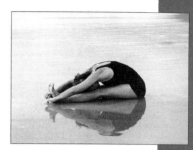

4. SUPTA PADANGHUSTASANA – LYING DOWN LEG STRETCH POSE

Lie on your back, bend your left leg, and place the left foot on the floor toward your left buttock. Inhale and raise your right leg, holding onto your foot with your right hand. Use a belt around the foot to hold onto if you can't reach with your hand. Moving with the breath, release into the stretch in the hamstring and hip areas by softening with each exhalation and allowing the leg to gently release forward and down. Hold for 5 to 10 breaths. Inhale to release and repeat on the other side.

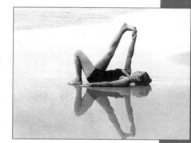

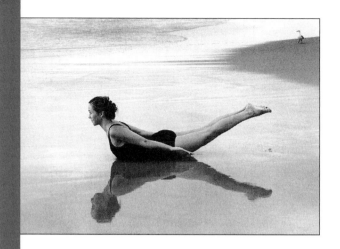

5. *SALABHASANA* – LOCUST POSE

Lie on your stomach and place your arms alongside your body, your palms facing upward. Rest your forehead on the floor. Inhale to raise your head, chest, shoulders, arms and legs off the floor, activating and strengthening your entire back; only the front of your torso and hips should be in contact with the floor. Focus forward and hold the position for 10 even breaths. Inhale to release down, rest and repeat.

Complete the sequence with *Halasana* (Chapter 5), Deep, full breathing (Chapter 2) and *Savasana* D (Chapter 4).

Cycling

A fluid body makes for a fluid ride. Correct positioning in the saddle and a relaxed upper body is the key. Balanced body tone is important. Unfortunately, cycling works some muscles of the body while others remain unused. The hips are constantly moving and if weak, the lower back compensates by bearing the strain. Counterbalance your cycling position with this sequence to stretch and lengthen your entire spine and your hips and legs, and to release tension in the neck, shoulders, hands and wrists.

Begin with Deep, full breathing (Chapter 2), East-west sequence (Chapter 6) and *Surya Namaskar* B (Chapter 6)

Before going on a ride, stretch your body and develop an even, flowing breath. Maintain this flow as you cycle.

1. GARUDASANA – EAGLE POSE

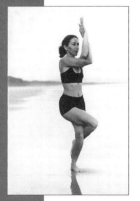

Stand with your feet together. Bend your knees and cross your right leg over the left, tucking your right foot behind your left ankle. Keeping your knees bent, raise your arms to shoulder height. Bend your forearms up to create a 90-degree angle. Cross your left arm over the right, bringing the left palm around to meet the right palm and stretching your hands and wrists. Keep your forearms moving away from your head and your eyes forward. Balance for 5 breaths and repeat on the other side.

2. ADHO MUKHA SVANASANA RESTING ON THE FOREARMS – DOWN FACE DOG POSE

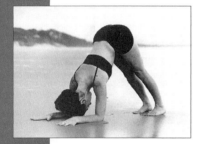

Kneel on the floor. Extend your arms out in front and step your feet back. Inhale to raise your hips and buttocks and straighten your legs, keeping your heels to the ground, hip-width apart. Keeping your forearms and palms firmly on the ground, lift your spine upward. Keeping eye focus toward your feet, hold for 5 to 10 deep, full breaths. Exhale to release down and rest.

3. URDHVA MUKHA SVANASANA – UP FACE DOG POSE

Lie on your stomach with your arms bent and the palms of your hands on the floor beside your shoulders and your legs extending away behind, the tops of your feet against the floor. Inhale and raise your head, torso and legs off the floor. Roll your shoulders back to open up your chest. Keep your legs and arms locked. Focus forward or gently drop your head back. Hold for 10 deep, full breaths, expanding the chest fully. Exhale to release down and rest.

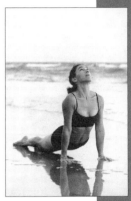

4. USTRASANA – CAMEL POSE

Kneel on the floor with your legs hip-width apart and hands on hips. Inhale and lift out from the waist and lower vertebrae. Exhale and slowly release your head back, bending your spine and moving your hips forward. If you have the flexibility, rest your hands on your feet behind you; if not, place a chair behind you with a bolster on it and, as you descend, rest your elbows and arms on the bolster. Hold for 5 to 10 breaths. Inhale to come up, releasing one hand at a time for support.

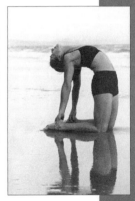

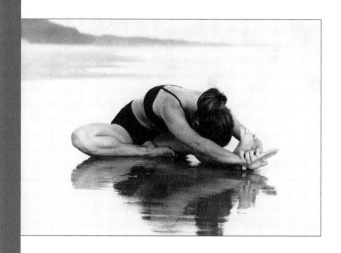

5. JANU SIRSASANA – HEAD TO KNEE POSE

Sit with your legs outstretched and bend your right leg up, placing the heel close to your groin, with the sole of your foot facing upward. Release the right knee down to the floor, opening up your right hip. Inhale and lift the front of your body. Exhale and extend forward and down to lie your torso over the length of your left leg, elongating the hamstrings and softening your back muscles. Breathe softly and fully for 5 breaths. Inhale, come up out of the posture, and repeat on the other side.

Complete this sequence with Cat curls (Chapter 6), Alternate-nostril breathing (Chapter 2) and *Savasana* C (Chapter 4).

Swimming and other water sports

Before you take the splash, take a deep breath and get into the flow with this pre-swim stretching sequence.

Yoga is the perfect partner for swimmers. It improves lung capacity, develops a flexible and strong body, and increases willpower, endurance levels and mental focus. Swimming requires even, focused breathing and body rhythm, which makes yoga the perfect preparation: it adds grace and flow to your style with the practice of deep, full, rhythmic breathing in the postures.

This sequence of postures stretches out the lower back and shoulder joints, and expands the chest, heart and lungs.

Begin with Deep, full breathing (Chapter 2), *Surya Namaskar* A (Chapter 6) and *Surya Namaskar* B (Chapter 6).

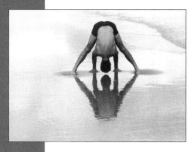

1. *PADOTTANASANA* I – FOOT-LEG EXTENSION POSE

Stand with your feet about five feet apart and your hands on your hips. Inhale and extend up and out from your waist. Exhale and slowly extend all the way forward and down, placing the palms of your hands on the floor between your feet. Contract and lift your front leg muscles, and lean forward into the balls of your feet, stretching the backs of your legs. Soften your spine, head and neck, keeping your shoulders lifted. Eye focus to the navel. Hold 5 to 10 even breaths through the nose. Inhale to come up.

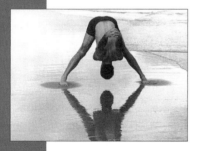

2. *PADOTTANASANA* III – FOOT-LEG EXTENSION POSE

Stand with your feet about five feet apart. Interlock your fingers behind you. Inhale and raise your arms, extending up and out from your waist. Exhale and bend at your hips, slowly bringing your arms over your head and your hands toward the ground. Lock your legs, lean forward into the balls of your feet and feel the stretch in your hamstrings. Soften your spine, head and neck, and release your shoulders. Hold for 5 to 10 even breaths through the nose. Inhale to come up.

3. URDHVA MUKHA SVANASANA –
UP FACE DOG POSE

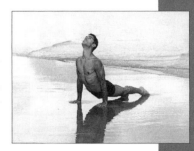

Lie on your stomach with your arms bent and the palms of your hands on the floor beside your shoulders and your legs extending away, the tops of your feet against the floor. Inhale and raise your head, torso and legs off the floor. Roll your shoulders back to open up your chest. Keep your legs and arms locked. Focus forward or gently drop your head back. Hold for 10 deep, full breaths, expanding the chest fully. Exhale to release down and rest.

4. ARDHA MATSYENDRASANA VARIATION –
HALF FISH LORD POSE

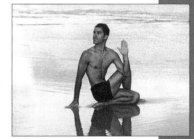

Sit with your legs extended out straight. Bend your left leg, placing the foot under the right leg and on the outside of the right buttock. Bend your right leg and place the right foot on the outside of your bent left knee. Place your left arm over your right knee. Inhale and turn to look over your right shoulder, placing your right hand behind you on the ground for support. Working in the pose, inhale to lift out from the waist, and exhale to twist and release deeper into the spine. After 5 full breaths, exhale to release and repeat on the opposite side.

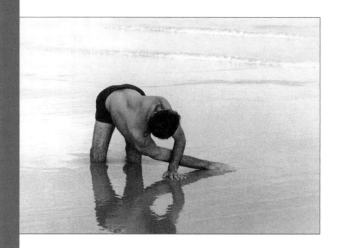

5. CAT SHOULDER STRETCH

Kneel on your hands and knees. Drop your right shoulder to the floor and, turning your head to look over your left shoulder, place your right arm under the left, reaching out the left. Feel the stretch in your right shoulder. Hold for 5 breaths, release and repeat with the left arm.

Complete the sequence with *Halasana* (Chapter 5), Preparation *Salamba Sarvangasana* (Chapter 5) and *Savasana* A (Chapter 4).

Tennis and squash

Swinging a racquet is a one-sided action that, if repeated, can throw out spinal muscles and build up just one side of the body. Balance your physical and mental self with these postures to elongate and align your muscles, strengthen your legs and back, and develop focus and mental power to promote skillful coordination and timing. Remain aware of your breathing and keep releasing any holding patterns.

Begin with Deep, full breathing (Chapter 2), East-west sequence (Chapter 6), and Forward hang (Chapter 5).

Be calm on the court by playing from your centerpoint, not just from your strong side, and develop inner strength and awareness.

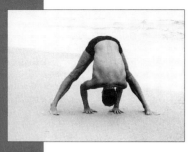

I. *PADOTTANASANA* I – FOOT-LEG EXTENSION POSE

Stand with your feet about five feet apart and your hands on your hips. Inhale and extend up and out from your waist. Exhale and slowly extend all the way forward and down, placing the palms of your hands on the floor between your feet. Contract and lift your front leg muscles, and lean forward into the balls of your feet, stretching your hamstrings. Soften your spine, head, neck and lift shoulders. Hold 5 to 10 even breaths through the nose. Inhale to come up.

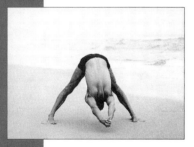

2. *PADOTTANASANA* III – FOOT-LEG EXTENSION POSE

Stand with your feet about five feet apart. Interlock your fingers behind you. Inhale and raise your arms, extending up and out from your waist. Exhale and bend at your hips, slowly bringing your arms over your head and your hands toward the ground. Lock your legs, lean forward into the balls of your feet and feel the stretch in your hamstrings. Soften your spine, head and neck, and release your shoulders. Hold for 5 to 10 even breaths through the nose. Inhale to come up.

3. GOMUKHASANA - COW HEAD POSE

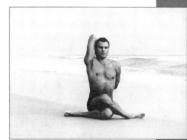

Kneel with your hands on the floor. Lean forward and cross your right leg over your left. Spread your feet away from your hips and sit between them on the floor. With your buttocks releasing down, bring your feet closer to your hips. Inhale and raise your right arm, bending your elbow and placing the palm of your hand down your back. Bring your left arm behind and interlock the fingers. Draw your right elbow back away from your head. Focus on releasing deeper into the shoulders and hips. Hold for 5 breaths, release and repeat on other side.

4. DHANURASANA - BOW POSE

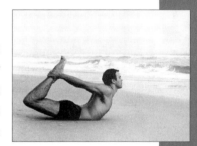

Lie on your stomach, bend your knees, lifting your feet behind you in the air, and press your pubis to the floor. Inhale and bring your hands back to hold your ankles while raising your head and chest off the ground. Focus on drawing your head upward, your legs together, opening up your shoulders and lifting your chest. Look forward and lightly squeeze the buttocks. Hold for 5 full breaths. Exhale to release down, rest and repeat twice.

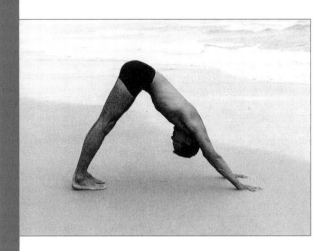

5. ADHO MUKHA SVANASANA – DOWN FACE DOG POSE

Kneel on the floor, extend your arms forward and step your feet back. Tucking your toes under, inhale to straighten your legs, raise your hips and buttocks, releasing your heels to the floor, hip-width apart. Soften your chest through your shoulders. Have a soft eye gaze in the direction of your feet. Hold for 5 to 10 breaths. Exhale as you release down, then rest.

Complete this sequence with Cat curls (Chapter 6), Alternate-nostril breathing (Chapter 2) and *Savasana* A (Chapter 4).

Golf

Golf is a healthy sport that develops concentration and inward focus as you aim the putts. However, it is also a one-sided action: swing after swing creates imbalance in the body. Correct alignment and breathing will increase your sense of physical balance, coordination and focus. Avoid muscular and spinal problems by taking the time to perform these stretching and strengthening postures before grabbing the clubs.

Begin with Deep, full breathing (Chapter 2), *Surya Namaskar A* (Chapter 6) and East-west sequence (Chapter 6).

This **balancing** sequence promotes **awareness** and many holes in one! Before you putt your next ball, get in touch with the breath and **align** yourself physically and **mentally**.

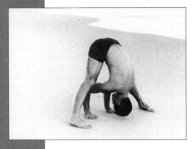

1. *PADOTTANASANA* I – FOOT-LEG EXTENSION POSE

Stand with your feet about five feet apart and your hands on your hips. Inhale and extend up and out from your waist. Exhale and slowly extend all the way forward and down, placing the palms of your hands on the floor between your feet. Contract and lift your front leg muscles, and lean forward into the balls of your feet, stretching your hamstrings. Soften your spine, head, neck and lift your shoulders. Hold 5 to 10 even breaths through the nose. Inhale to come up.

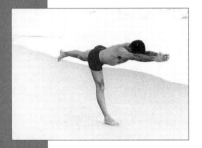

2. *VIRABHADRASANA* III – WARRIOR POSE

Stand upright then step your right foot forward about five feet. Inhale and lift out from your waist. Exhale, bend your right knee and lean over your right leg, raising your left foot off the ground behind you. Extend your arms forward and lift your back leg in line with your torso. Find your balance and straighten the standing leg. Stay focusing forward in this strengthening and balancing posture for 5 breaths. Inhale to release to standing, and repeat on the other side.

3. PARIGHASANA – GATE POSE

Kneel on the floor and place your hands on your hips. Exhale and extend your right leg out to the right, keeping the foot in line with your hip. Place your right hand on your right leg, down toward the foot. Inhale and extend out from the waist, raising your left arm. Exhale and extend your left arm over your head, the palm facing down. Tuck in your chin and look up to the left hand. Keep the left hip above the left knee. Breathe into the side of your torso as you release in the stretch for 5 breaths. Inhale to release and repeat on the other side.

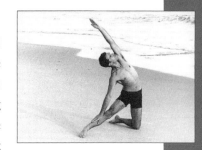

4. URDHVA MUKHA SVANASANA – UP FACE DOG POSE

Lie on your stomach with your arms bent and the palms of your hands on the floor beside your shoulders and your legs extending away, with the tops of your feet on the floor. Inhale and raise your head, torso and legs off the floor. Roll your shoulders back to open up your chest. Keep your legs and arms locked. Focus forward or gently drop your head back. Hold for 10 deep, full breaths, expanding the chest fully. Exhale to release down and rest.

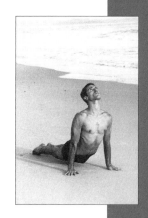

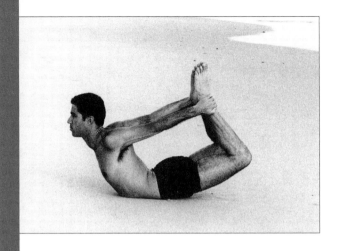

5. *DHANURASANA* – BOW POSE

Lie on your stomach, bend your knees, lifting your feet behind you in the air, and press your pubis to the floor. Inhale and bring your hands back to hold your ankles while raising your head and chest off the ground. Focus on drawing your head upward, your knees together, opening up your shoulders and lifting your chest. Look forward and lightly squeeze the buttocks. Hold for 5 full breaths. Exhale to release down, rest and repeat twice.

Complete this sequence with Cat curls (Chapter 6), Alternate-nostril breathing (Chapter 2) and *Savasana* B (Chapter 4).

Basketball
and volleyball

Ball sports develop a strong body and good coordination skills. With the main point of focus being the ball, you will benefit from yoga postures that enhance performance and develop concentration and focus. Team sports can be quite stressful at times, especially when playing an important game. To counteract this, strengthen your legs and back and reduce the build up of tension in the shoulders with this sequence. And remember to keep your arms fluid and your hands relaxed on the ball.

Begin with Deep, full breathing (Chapter 2), Alternate-nostril breathing (Chapter 2) and *Surya Namaskar A* (Chapter 6).

Relax the whole body and develop concentration and awareness by remaining focused on the inhalation and exhalation throughout the sequence and the game!

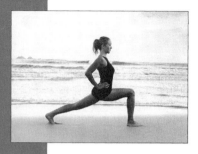

1. LEG LUNGE

Begin from a kneeling position, place your hands on your hips and step your right foot forward. Inhale and lift out from your waist. Exhale and lift your left knee and leg off the ground. Keeping your right knee bent and your thigh at a 90-degree angle, drop your left knee down toward the floor to create a stretch in the left quadriceps and the front of the hip. Lift up and down for 5 breaths, releasing further with each exhalation. Inhale to come out of the position, return to kneeling and repeat on the left side.

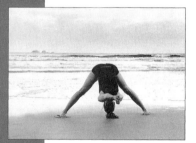

2. *PADOTTANASANA* III – FOOT-LEG EXTENSION POSE

Stand with your feet about five feet apart. Interlock your fingers behind you. Inhale and raise your arms, extending up and out from your waist. Exhale and bend at your hips, slowly bringing your arms over your head and your hands toward the ground. Lock your legs, lean forward into the balls of your feet and feel the stretch in your hamstrings. Soften your spine, head and neck, and release your shoulders. Hold for 5 to 10 even breaths through the nose. Inhale to come up.

3. SALABHASANA – LOCUST POSE

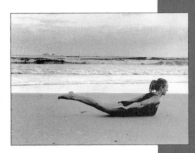

Lie on your stomach and place your arms alongside your body, your palms facing upward. Rest your forehead on the floor. Inhale to raise your head, chest, arms, shoulders and legs off the floor, activating and strengthening your entire back; only the front of your torso and hips are in contact with the floor. Focus forward and hold the position for 10 even breaths. Inhale to release down, rest and repeat.

4. URDHVA MUKHA SVANASANA – UP FACE DOG POSE

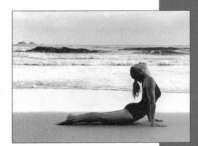

Lie on your stomach with your arms bent and the palms of your hands on the floor beside your shoulders and your legs extending away, with the tops of your feet on the floor. Inhale and raise your head, torso and hips off the floor. Roll your shoulders back to open up your chest. Keep your legs and arms locked. Focus forward or gently drop your head back. Hold for 10 deep, full breaths, expanding the chest fully. Exhale to release down and rest.

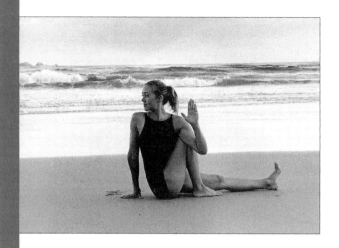

5. *MARICYASANA* TWIST – INDIAN SAGE POSE

Sit with your legs outstretched and bend your right leg, placing your foot on the floor near your groin so that your thigh is touching your abdomen. Place your right hand on the floor behind your right hip. Lock your left arm in front of your right knee, pressing your knee into your arm. Inhale and lift up from your hips, thinning your waist. Exhale and twist to look over your right shoulder. Keep your left leg straight in front and the muscles activated. Release into the twist for 5 breaths. Exhale to come back to center, and repeat on the other side.

Complete the sequence with East-west sequence (Chapter 6), Supported *Salamba Sarvangasana* (Chapter 5) and *Savasana* A (Chapter 4).

Skiing and snowboarding

Good balance is the key for skiers and boarders because in maintaining balance, the center point of gravity is always shifting and the body is therefore having to constantly realign. This sequence teaches balance, stretches the legs and strengthens the back. Having a strong and flexible physical body will add joy to the feeling of freedom that skiing or boarding gives. They are sports that require 100 percent strength from the start to the finish of the run.

Begin with Deep, full breathing (Chapter 2), *Surya Namaskar A* (Chapter 6), and *Surya Namaskar* C (Chapter 6).

When we are completely **present** in the moment, there is no thought and **no fear**. Being on the slopes and in this **no-mind** state is the experience that brings enthusiasts back season after season.

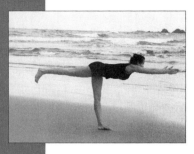

1. *VIRABHADRASANA* III – WARRIOR POSE

Stand upright then step your right foot forward about five feet. Inhale and lift out from your waist. Exhale, bend your right knee and lean over your right leg, raising your left foot off the ground behind you. Extend your arms forward and lift your back leg in line with your torso. Find your balance and straighten the standing leg. Stay focusing forward in this strengthening and balancing posture for 5 breaths. Inhale to release to standing, and repeat on the other side.

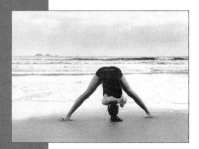

2. *PADOTTANASANA* III – FOOT-LEG EXTENSION POSE

Stand with your feet about five feet apart. Interlock your fingers behind you. Inhale and raise your arms, extending up and out from your waist. Exhale and bend at your hips, slowly bringing your arms over your head and your hands toward the ground. Lock your legs, lean forward into the balls of your feet and feel the stretch in your hamstrings. Soften your spine, head and neck, and release your shoulders. Hold for 5 to 10 even breaths through the nose. Inhale to come up.

3. URDHVA MUKHA SVANASANA –
UP FACE DOG POSE

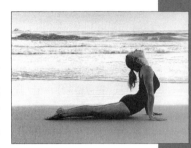

Lie on your stomach with your arms bent and the palms of your hands on the floor beside your shoulders and your legs extending away, with the tops of your feet on the floor. Inhale and raise your head, torso and hips off the floor. Roll your shoulders back to open up your chest. Keep your legs and arms locked. Focus forward or gently drop your head back. Hold for 10 deep, full breaths, expanding the chest fully. Exhale to release down and rest.

4. USTRASANA – CAMEL POSE

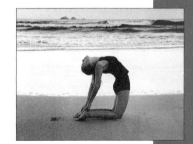

Kneel on the floor with your legs hip-width apart and hands on hips. Inhale and lift out from the waist and lower vertebrae. Exhale and slowly release your head back, bending your spine and pushing your hips forward. If you have the flexibility, rest your hands on your feet behind you; if not, place a chair behind you with a bolster on it and, as you descend, rest your elbows and arms on the bolster. Hold for 5 to 10 breaths. Inhale to come up, releasing one hand at a time for support.

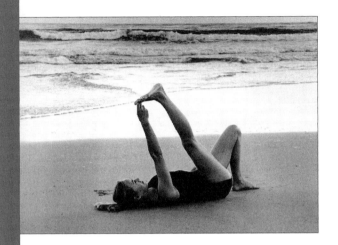

5. SUPTA PADANGHUSTASANA – LYING DOWN LEG STRETCH POSE

Lie on your back, bend your left leg, and place the left foot on the floor toward your left hip. Inhale and raise your right leg, holding onto your foot with your right hand. Loop a belt around your foot if you can't reach. Moving with the breath, release into the stretch in the hamstring and hip areas by softening with each exhalation and allowing the leg to gently release forward and down. Hold for 5 to 10 breaths. Inhale to release and repeat on the other side.

Complete this sequence with Chair rest (Chapter 5), Alternate-nostril breathing (Chapter 2) and *Savasana* C (Chapter 4).

Surfing and boogie boarding

Surfing requires skill and strength. A supple body and good balance are essential. Lots of energy is needed to get out to the waves, and then the maneuvering techniques begin! More and more surfers are limbering up before they hit the waves to increase mobility and endurance, and to avoid soft tissue damage from sudden, irregular movements. Yoga also increases lung capacity, which can be a vital asset when you find yourself plunged into the ocean depths.

Begin with Deep, full breathing (Chapter 2), Cat curls (Chapter 6) and *Surya Namaskar* A (Chapter 6).

Being flexible and balanced in the water and on the board helps maintain those exhilarating rides, allowing you to be fluid and focused on the journey.

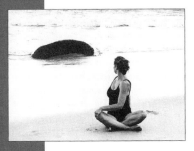

1. SUKHASANA TWIST – HAPPY TWIST POSE

Sit in an easy cross-legged position. Place your left hand onto your right knee and your right hand behind you on the floor. Inhale to lift out from your waist, and exhale to twist and look over your right shoulder. Inhale to lift and exhale to twist. Exhale, release to the center, then twist to the left side, focusing on releasing tension from your shoulders, spine and hips with each exhalation. After 5 breaths, release, and come back to center.

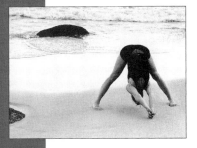

2. PADOTTANASANA III – FOOT-LEG EXTENSION POSE

Stand with your feet about five feet apart. Interlock your fingers behind you. Inhale and raise your arms, extending up and out from your waist. Exhale and bend at your hips, slowly bringing your arms over your head and your hands toward the ground. Lock your legs, lean forward into the balls of your feet and feel the stretch in your hamstrings. Soften your spine, head and neck, and release your shoulders. Hold for 5 to 10 even breaths through the nose. Inhale to come up.

3. URDHVA MUKHA SVANASANA –
UP FACE DOG POSE

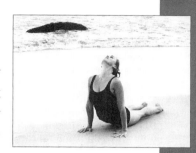

Lie on your stomach with your arms bent and the palms of your hands on the floor beside your shoulders and your legs extending away, with the tops of your feet on the floor. Inhale and raise your head, torso and legs off the floor. Roll your shoulders back to open up your chest. Keep your legs and arms locked. Focus forward or gently drop your head back. Hold for 10 deep, full breaths, expanding the chest fully. Exhale to release down and rest.

4. HIP STRETCH

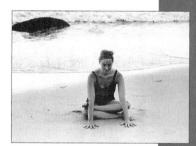

Sit on the floor with your legs outstretched. Bend your right knee and rest it on the floor away from your torso. Bring your left foot to rest on the right knee, and the left knee to rest on your right foot. Inhale and, with your hands on the floor in front of you, exhale and lean forward, releasing the left knee down to stretch open the left hip muscles. Hold for a few breaths and repeat on the other side.

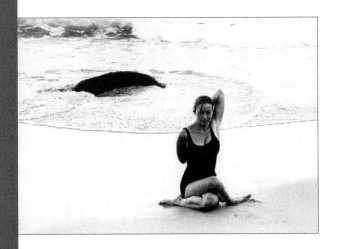

5. GOMUKHASANA – COW HEAD POSE

Kneel with your hands on the floor. Lean forward and cross your right leg over your left. Spread your feet away from your hips and sit between them on the floor. With your buttocks releasing down, bring your feet closer to your hips. Inhale and raise your left arm, bending your elbow and placing the palm of your hand down your back behind your head. Bring your right arm behind and interlock the fingers. Draw your left elbow back away from your head. Focus on releasing deeper into the shoulders and hips. Hold for 5 breaths, release and repeat on other side.

Complete the sequence with Supported shoulder stand (Chapter 5), Deep, full breathing (Chapter 2) and *Savasana* A (Chapter 4).

Weightlifting

More and more body builders are awakening to the great benefits of yoga for increased mental power and focus, and the ability to relax the nervous system at will. Body builders who are developing and strengthening specific muscle groups can practice before, during or after training to relax and release tension and help make the short, intense lifts more fluid. A flexible yoga body decreases the likelihood of muscle strain. Practice deep, full breathing to release unwanted tightness and tension.

Begin with Deep, full breathing (Chapter 2), Cat curls (Chapter 6) and *Surya Namaskar* B (Chapter 6).

Bring some softness and relaxation into your training: release any holding in the body and mind and develop an even breathing pattern, flexibility, endurance and focus.

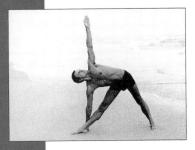

1. *TRIKONASANA* – TRIANGLE POSE

Stand with your feet about four feet apart. Turn your right foot out 90 degrees and the left foot in 45 degrees. Extend your arms out to the sides at shoulder height. Inhale and extend the right side of your torso over to the right. Exhale and place your right hand onto your right ankle or on the floor. Tuck your chin in, extend your left arm up and turn to look beyond the fingertips of your left hand. Keep the muscles of your legs and arms activated, and the left hip opening. Inhale to release and bring yourself up. Exhale to turn and repeat on the other side.

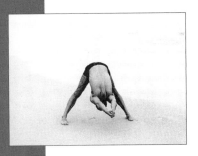

2. *PADOTTANASANA* III – FOOT-LEG EXTENSION POSE

Stand with your feet about five feet apart. Interlock your fingers behind you. Inhale and raise your arms, extending up and out from your waist. Exhale and bend at your hips, slowly bringing your arms over your head and your hands toward the ground. Lock your legs, lean forward into the balls of your feet and feel the stretch in your hamstrings. Soften your spine, head and neck, and release your shoulders. Hold for 5 to 10 even breaths through the nose. Inhale to come up.

3. CAT SHOULDER STRETCH

Kneel on your hands and knees. Drop your right shoulder to the floor and, turning your head to look over your left shoulder, place your right arm under the left, reaching out the left. Feel the stretch in your right shoulder. Hold for 5 breaths, release and repeat with the left arm.

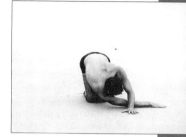

4. *BADDHA KONASANA* – BOUND ANGLE POSE

Sit on the floor with the soles of your feet together. Interlock your fingers around your toes and lift out from your lower back. Let your knees relax to the floor and the muscles around your hips soften. Roll your shoulders down and back, and lift your torso to open the chest. Breathe into the opening around your hips, softening with each exhalation. Hold for 10 deep, full breaths then release.

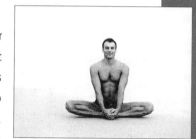

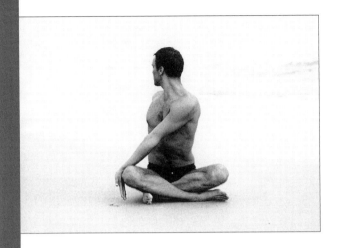

5. SUKHASANA TWIST – HAPPY TWIST POSE

Sit in an easy cross-legged position. With your back straight, place your left hand onto your right knee and your right hand behind you on the floor. Inhale to lift out from your waist, and exhale to twist and look over your right shoulder. Inhale to lift out and exhale to twist for 5 breaths. Exhale to release to the center, then twist to the left side, focusing on releasing tension from your shoulders and hips with each exhalation. After 5 breaths, release, and come back to center.

Complete this sequence with a Forward rest (Chapter 11), Alternate-nostril breathing (Chapter 2) and *Savasana* C (Chapter 4).

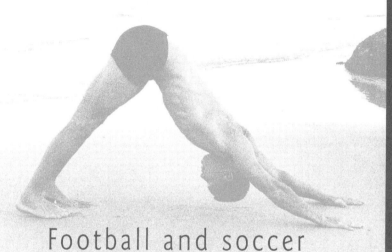

Football and soccer

These high-energy games require endurance and inner and outer strength. Regular yoga practice builds stamina, mobility and willpower, encourages correct breathing, and keeps you focused and on the move for longer. Practice this sequence to loosen up, prevent leg and back injuries and improve breathing.

Begin with Deep, full breathing (Chapter 2), Alternate-nostril breathing (Chapter 2) and *Surya Namaskar* A (Chapter 6).

Balance out these leg-focused sports with this upper-body sequence to promote **suppleness** and **fluidity** in the back, chest and shoulders.

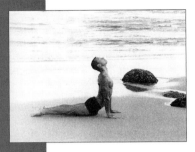

1. URDHVA MUKHA SVANASANA –
UP FACE DOG POSE

Lie on your stomach with your arms bent and the palms of your hands on the floor beside your shoulders and your legs extending away, with the tops of your feet on the floor. Inhale and raise your head, torso and legs off the floor. Roll your shoulders back to open up your chest. Keep your legs and arms locked. Focus forward or gently drop your head back. Hold for 10 deep, full breaths, expanding the chest fully. Exhale to release down and rest.

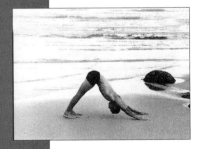

2. ADHO MUKHA SVANASANA –
DOWN FACE DOG POSE

Kneel on the floor, extend your arms forward and step your feet back. Tucking your toes under, straighten your legs, lift your hips and buttocks, releasing your heels to the floor, hip-width apart. Soften your chest through your shoulders. Have a soft eye gaze in the direction of your feet. Hold for 5 to 10 breaths. Exhale as you release down, then rest.

3. LEG LUNGE

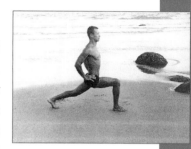

Begin from a kneeling position, place your hands on your hips and step your right foot forward. Inhale and lift out from your waist. Exhale and lift your left knee and leg off the ground. Keeping your right knee bent and your thigh at a 90-degree angle, drop your left knee down toward the floor to create a stretch in the left quadriceps and the front of the hip. Lift up and down for 5 breaths, releasing further with each exhalation. Inhale to come out of the position, return to kneeling and repeat on the left side.

4. *SUPTA PADANGHUSTASANA –* LYING DOWN LEG STRETCH POSE

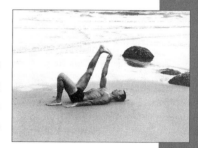

Lie on your back, bend your left leg, and place the left foot on the floor toward your left hip. Inhale and raise your right leg, holding onto your foot with your right hand. Use a belt around the foot to hold onto if you cannot reach. Moving with the breath, release into the stretch in the hamstring and hip areas by softening with each exhalation and allowing the leg to gently release forward and down. Hold for 5 to 10 breaths. Inhale to release and repeat on the other side.

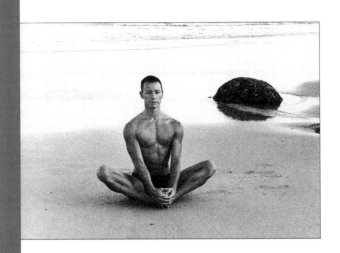

5. BADDHA KONASANA – BOUND ANGLE POSE

Sit on the floor with the soles of your feet together. Interlock your fingers around your toes and lift out from your lower back. Let your knees relax to the floor and the muscles around your hips soften. Roll your shoulders down and back, and lift your torso to open the chest. Breathe into the opening around your hips, softening with each exhalation. Hold for 10 deep, full breaths then release.

Complete this sequence with the East-west sequence (Chapter 6), Meditation (Chapter 3) and *Savasana* D (Chapter 4).

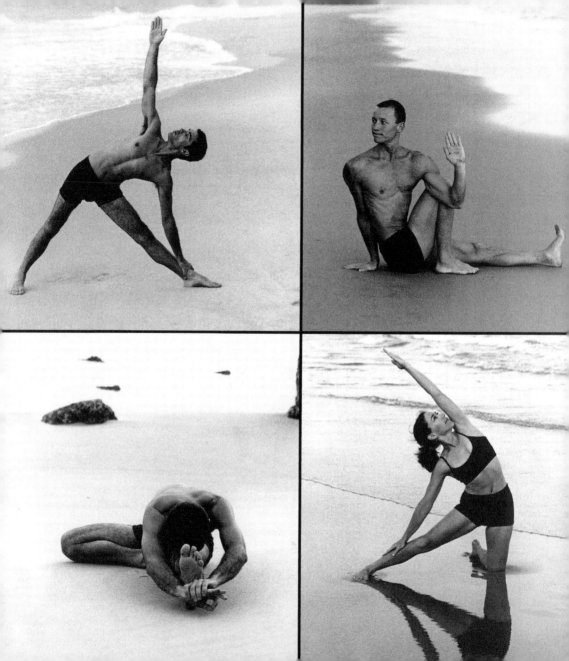

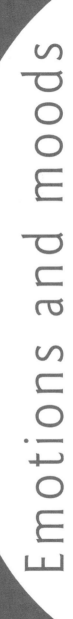

Emotions and moods

Yoga is a path of personal insight, change and growth – on physical, mental, emotional and spiritual levels. Yoga practice releases the body and frees the mind. Being aware in the postures is a journey into the self. The postures open tight areas of the body, massage deep into the organs and cleanse, stirring up and releasing stored emotions.

Become aware of the different effects postures have on your moods and emotions. Practice hip-opening positions to release sexual tension; forward bends to cool and give mental calm and peace of mind; backward bends to expand the heart, stimulate open communication and release fear; and twisting postures to clear away negative feelings.

Use your breathe. When you experience a rush of emotion, you can enhance your experience of the emotion by drawing it in with an inhalation of breath, or you can simply let it go by consciously breathing it out on the exhalation breathe.

Practice breath awareness throughout the day to provide emotional calm and to release negative, unwanted emotions. We all have the power to choose how we react to situations and how we feel. Use your breath as a tool to enjoy life.

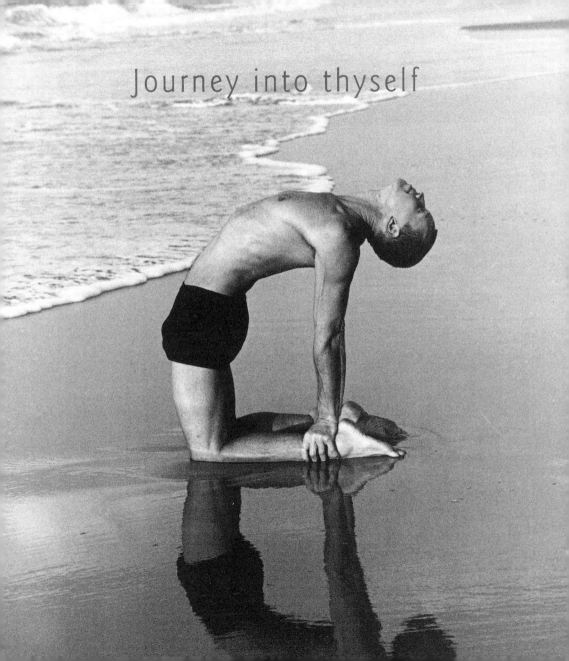

Journey into thyself

Preparing for work

Whether working from home or elsewhere, it pays to prepare yourself mentally and physically for the day. With more blood and therefore oxygen flowing throughout your body and to the brain, your mind is less likely to wander and you're more able to focus on the job at hand. Feeling good about yourself goes hand in hand with looking after yourself. Practice this sequence to get you in the mood for work and be inspired!

Begin with Deep, full breathing (Chapter 2), *Surya Namaskar* A (Chapter 6) and *Surya Namaskar* B (Chapter 6).

Make your work time enjoyable and productive with a healthy body and mind that is focused, inspired and energized.

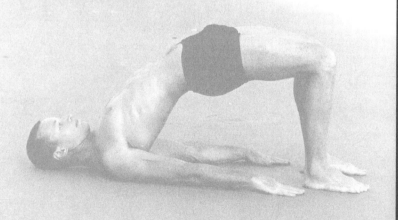

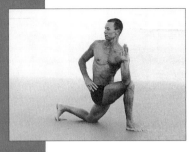

1. PARIVRTTA PARSVAKONASANA VARIATION – REVOLVED SIDEWAYS ANGLE POSE

From a standing position, step your right foot forward about five feet and, squaring your hips to the front, lunge forward on the right leg into a right angle. Rest your left knee on the floor. Exhale and turn to look over your right shoulder while placing your left hand on the floor beside your right foot. Rest your right hand on your right hip. Inhale to lift out from your waist, then exhale to twist further to the right. Hold for 5 breaths. Inhale to release out of the pose and change sides.

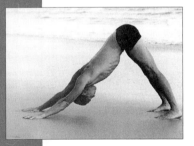

2. ADHO MUKHA SVANASANA – DOWN FACE DOG POSE

Kneel on the floor, extend your arms forward and step your feet back. Tucking your toes under, inhale to straighten your legs, lift your hips and buttocks, releasing your heels to the floor, hip-width apart. Soften your chest through your shoulders. Have a soft eye gaze in the direction of your feet. Hold for 5 to 10 breaths. Exhale as you release down, then rest.

3. NAVASANA – BOAT POSE

Sit on the floor and find your balance forward on your sitting bones. Move around until you feel centered. Bend and raise your legs halfway in toward your chest, and extend your arms out parallel to your lower legs. Lift your lower back in and up so that your spine isn't collapsing. Hold for 5 to 10 breaths, release, rest and repeat twice. If you have the strength, aim to straighten your legs.

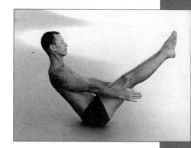

4. MINI BACKBEND

Lie on your back and bend your legs, placing your feet next to your buttocks, hip-width apart. Extend your arms alongside your body with the palms facing down. Exhale and slowly roll up off the floor, getting in touch with each vertebra as you do, first lifting your buttocks, then lower back, middle back and chest to form a backward arch. Keep your shoulders on the floor. Squeeze your buttocks together and lift your hips high. Hold for 5 breaths, release gently, rest and repeat.

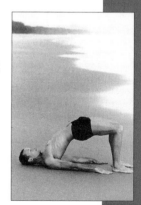

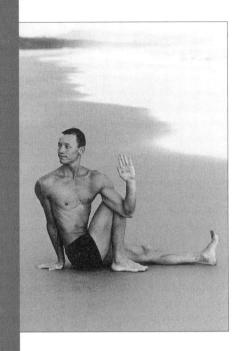

5. *MARICYASANA* TWIST – INDIAN SAGE POSE

Sit with your legs outstretched and bend your right leg, placing your foot on the floor near your groin so that your thigh is touching your abdomen. Place your right hand on the floor behind your right hip. Lock your left arm in front of your right knee, pressing your knee into your arm. Inhale and lift up from your hips, thinning your waist. Exhale and twist to look over your right shoulder. Keep your left leg straight in front and the muscles activated. Release into the twist for 5 breaths. Release, come back to center, and repeat on the other side.

Complete the sequence with Cat curls (Chapter 6), *Salamba Sarvangasana* (Chapter 5) and *Savasana* A (Chapter 4).

Relaxing after a busy day

When feeling scattered after a big day, spend some time rebalancing your body, mind and spirit. These stress-releasing, cleansing and centering postures help overcome exhaustion and bring us back to the here and now. Create some space and peace of mind to embrace the night.

Begin with Meditation (Chapter 3), Deep, full breathing (Chapter 2) and Forward hang (Chapter 5).

Ask yourself how you **feel** now, and how you know you'll **feel** after some yoga practice. You'll soon find yourself in position and ready to **renew** your whole being.

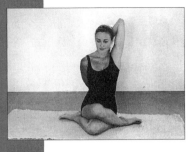

1. GOMUKHASANA – COW HEAD POSE

Kneel with your hands on the floor. Lean forward and cross your right leg over your left. Spread your feet away from your hips and sit between them on the floor. With your buttocks releasing down, bring your feet closer to your hips. Inhale and raise your left arm, bending your elbow and placing the palm of your hand down your back behind your head. Bring your right arm behind your back and interlock the fingers of both hands. Draw your left elbow away from your head. Focus on releasing deeper into the shoulders and hips. Hold for 5 breaths, release and repeat on other side.

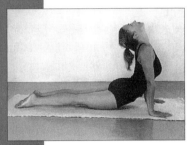

2. URDHVA MUKHA SVANASANA – UP FACE DOG POSE

Lie on your stomach with your arms bent and the palms of your hands on the floor beside your shoulders and your legs extending away, with the tops of your feet on the floor. Inhale and raise your head, torso and hips off the floor. Roll your shoulders back to open up your chest. Keep your legs and arms locked. Focus forward or gently drop your head back. Hold for 10 deep, full breaths, expanding the chest fully. Exhale to release down and rest.

3. *ADHO MUKHA SVANASANA* –
DOWN FACE DOG POSE

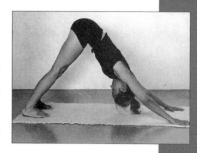

Kneel on the floor, extend your arms forward and step your feet back. Tucking your toes under, inhale to straighten your legs, raise your hips and buttocks, releasing your heels to the floor, hip-width apart. Soften your chest through your shoulders. Have a soft eye gaze in the direction of your feet. Hold for 5 to 10 breaths. Exhale as you release down, then rest.

4. *SUPTA BADDHA KONASANA*
LYING OVER A BOLSTER LENGTHWISE –
SUPINE BOUND ANGLE POSE

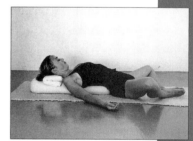

Sit with outstretched legs, a bolster or folded blankets extending lengthwise behind you. With your buttocks on the floor and your lower back touching the end of the bolster, exhale and lie back over the bolster, resting your head and upper back on it. Tuck in your chin and extend your arms to the sides. Bring the soles of your feet together, allowing your legs to splay open and your knees to drop to the floor. Close your eyes and focus on breathing fully and opening out your chest, lungs and heart. Rest in this position for 5 to 10 minutes.

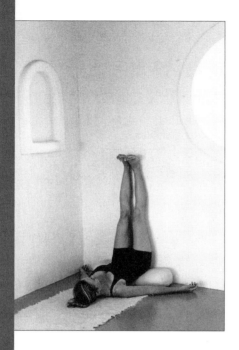

5. VIPARITA KARANI – INVERTED PRACTICE

Place a bolster or some folded blankets next to a wall. Lie with your legs up the wall, your hips and pelvis elevated on the bolster so that they are higher than your heart. Relax your upper back, shoulders, neck and head on the floor, and relax your arms on the floor to your sides, palms facing up. Rest in this gentle, relaxed, inverted position for 5 to 10 minutes.

Complete this sequence with *Sarvangasana* (Chapter 5), Alternate-nostril breathing (Chapter 2) and *Savasana* C (Chapter 4).

Being present in the moment

Feeling alive and at one with the moment is one of the main benefits of yoga practice. Relieving the physical body of stress, calming the mind's chatter and focusing on the breath all bring us into a mindful and present state of being. Practice with the intention to enrich your life.

Begin with Deep, full breathing (Chapter 2), Cat curls (Chapter 6) and *Surya Namaskar* A (Chapter 6).

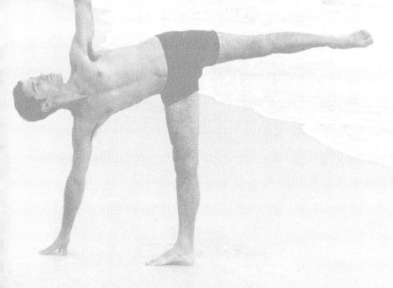

Enhance your be-ing-ness and presence in the moment with these balancing and focusing postures.

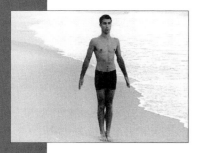

I. *TADASANA* – MOUNTAIN POSE

Stand with your feet together and your arms by your sides. Get in touch with your center and activate your whole body. Be in one straight line with your toes and the soles of your feet spread wide, your inner arches lifting, leg muscles contracting upward, buttocks slightly tucked under, your spine extending upward. Your shoulders rolling down and back and your chest open, activate your arms and gaze softly forward. Focus on inhaling and exhaling fully for 10 breaths.

2. *VRKSASANA* – TREE POSE

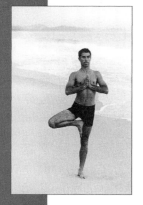

Begin in *Tadasana* (above), then bend your right leg, placing your right foot against your left thigh so it feels locked in. Move your right knee back to open your hip. Keep the muscles of your left leg activated and lifting. Center your bodyweight so that you aren't leaning on your standing leg too much. Place your hands in prayer position in front of your heart center. Roll your shoulders down and back to open your chest. Relax your facial muscles and gaze softly at a point in front at eye level. Hold for 5 full breaths. Exhale to release your leg and change sides.

3. *TRIKONASANA* – TRIANGLE POSE

Stand with your feet about four feet apart. Turn your right foot out 90 degrees and the left foot in 45 degrees. Extend your arms out to the sides at shoulder height. Inhale and lengthen your right arm and the right side of your torso over to the right. Exhale and place your right hand onto your right ankle. Tuck your chin in, extend your left arm up and turn to look beyond the fingertips of your left hand. Keep the muscles of your legs and arms activated and the left hip opening. Inhale to release and bring yourself up. Exhale to turn and repeat on the other side.

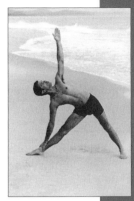

4. *ARDHA CHANDRASANA* – HALF MOON POSE

From *Trikonasana* (above), exhale as you bend your right knee and bring your right hand to the floor in front of your foot. Straighten your right leg as you raise your left leg up so the two legs form a right angle. Rotate your left hip around and back, activating the leg muscles for balance and strengthening. When you find your balance, raise your left arm straight up. Tuck your chin in and turn to look up and beyond your outstretched fingers or look to the floor. Hold for 5 to 10 focused breaths. Inhale to release to standing via *Trikonasana*. Repeat on the other side.

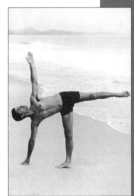

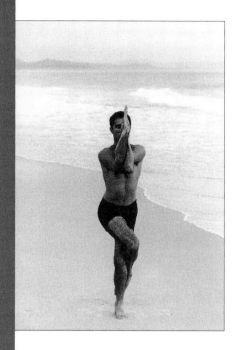

5. GARUDASANA - EAGLE POSE

Stand with your feet together. Bend your knees and cross your right leg over the left, tucking your right foot behind your left ankle. Keeping your knees bent, raise your arms to shoulder height. Bend your forearms up to create a 90-degree angle. Cross your left arm over the right, bringing the left palm around to meet the right palm, stretching your hands and wrists. Keep your forearms moving away from your head and open out your shoulders.

Complete the sequence with Alternate-nostril breathing (Chapter 2), Meditation (Chapter 3) and *Savasana* A (Chapter 4).

Releasing anger, fear and frustration

Help release these emotions from your mind and body with dynamic postures that cleanse the liver and other organs – dispelling negativity and making way for new beginnings. Maintain breath awareness to remove your focus from your troubles and to return to a space of clarity, inner calm and love.

Begin with Deep, full breathing (Chapter 2), East-west sequence (Chapter 6) and *Surya Namaskar* B (Chapter 6).

Practice this sequence with **deep** breathing to **cleanse** the organs and **release** stored fear and anger.

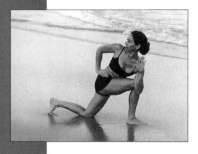

1. PARIVRTTA PARSVAKONASANA VARIATION – REVOLVED SIDEWAYS ANGLE POSE

From a standing position, step your right foot forward about five feet and, squaring your hips to the front, lunge forward on the right leg into a right angle. Rest your left knee on the floor. Exhale and turn to look over your right shoulder while placing your left hand over your right knee. Rest your right hand on your right hip. Inhale to lift out from your waist, then exhale to twist further to the right. Hold for 5 breaths. Inhale to release out of the pose and change sides.

2. PARIGHASANA – GATE POSE

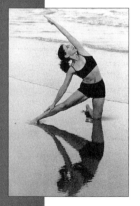

Kneel on the floor and place your hands on your hips. Exhale and extend your right leg out to the right, keeping the foot in line with your hip. Place your right hand on your right leg, down toward the foot. Inhale and extend out from the waist, raising your left arm. Exhale and extend your left arm over your head, the palm facing down. Tuck in your chin and look up to the left hand. Keep the left hip above the left knee. Breathe into the side of your torso as you release in the stretch for 5 breaths. Inhale to come up and repeat on the other side.

3. *MARICYASANA* TWIST – INDIAN SAGE POSE

Sit with your legs outstretched and bend your right leg, placing your foot on the floor near your groin so that your thigh is touching your abdomen. Place your right hand on the floor behind your right hip. Lock your left arm in front of your right knee, pressing your knee into your arm. Inhale and lift up from your hips, thinning your waist. Exhale and twist to look over your right shoulder. Keep your left leg straight in front and the muscles activated. Release into the twist for 5 breaths. Release, come back to center, and repeat on the other side.

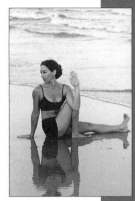

4. *ARDHA MATSYENDRASANA* VARIATION – HALF FISH LORD POSE

Sit with your legs extended out straight. Bend your left leg and place your left foot beside your right buttock. Bend your right leg and place the right foot on the outside of your bent left knee. Place your left arm over your right knee. Inhale and turn to look over your right shoulder, placing your right hand behind you on the ground for support. Working in the pose, inhale to lift out from the waist, and exhale to twist and release deeper into the spine. After 5 full breaths, exhale to release and repeat on the opposite side.

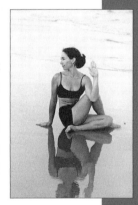

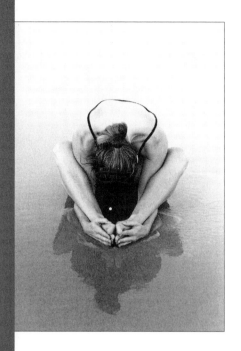

5. *KURMASANA* VARIATION – TORTOISE POSE

Sitting with the soles of your feet together, place your hands under your knees and slide your feet forward. Let your torso and head come down, and bring your hands around to meet your feet. Hang forward, relaxing your head, shoulders and spine. Hold the position for 10 full breaths. Inhale to come up slowly.

Complete this sequence with Supported *Halasana* (Chapter 5), Meditation (Chapter 3) and *Savasana* D (Chapter 4).

Calming the mind

A hyperactive mind, overloaded with thoughts, plans and decisions, can lead to anxiety and other problems. Find inner calm by returning to your center – the point between activity and inactivity, stress and calm. Learn to return to this centerpoint at will by practicing yoga postures, breath awareness and meditation.

Begin with Deep, full breathing (Chapter 2), Cat curls (Chapter 6) and Forward hang (Chapter 5).

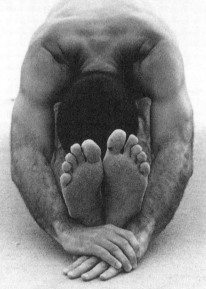

Find your point of **balance** and mental **calm** within the practice of these **nurturing** postures.

1. *VIRASANA* – HERO POSE

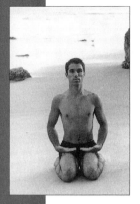

Sit with your buttocks on your ankles, then slide your heels out to the sides so your buttocks release to the ground and you are sitting between your heels. At this point, decide whether you will need to sit on some blankets to relieve any tightness in your legs, knees or ankles. Draw your knees in toward each other. Stretch the sides of your torso upward. Roll back your shoulders and open your chest. Rest the backs of your hands on your knees. Relax here for 5 breaths with soft eye gaze forward.

2. *JANU SIRSASANA* – HEAD TO KNEE POSE

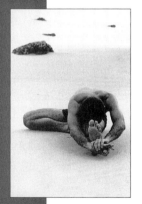

Sit with your legs outstretched and bend your right leg up, placing the heel close to your groin, with the sole of your foot facing upward. Release the right knee down to the floor, opening up your right hip. Inhale and lift the front of your body. Exhale and extend forward and down to lie your torso over the length of your left leg, elongating the hamstrings and loosening your back muscles. Breathe softly and fully for 5 breaths. Inhale, come up out of the posture, and repeat on the other side. Use a belt around your foot and keep your back straight if you can't rest forward.

3. *PASCIMOTTANASANA* – BACK EXTENSION POSE

Sit on the floor with your legs extended out straight in front and activated. Roll onto your sitting bones, then tilt your pelvis forward. Inhale, lift and extend your pubis, stomach and chest, then exhale to release down, lying forward and holding onto the outsides of your feet or wrapping your hands around your feet. Inhale to release up.

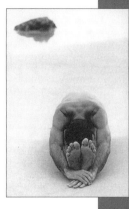

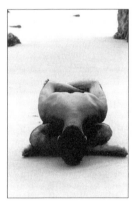

4. FORWARD *SUKHASANA*

Sit in an easy cross-legged position. Fold your arms behind your back, bringing your thumbs into the crease of the opposite elbow. Inhale, lifting out from the waist. Exhale to extend and release forward and down. Rest your forehead on the floor or a bolster. Hold for 10 full breaths. Inhale to release up.

5. *KURMASANA* VARIATION – TORTOISE POSE

Sitting with the soles of your feet together, place your hands under your knees and slide your feet forward. Let your torso and head come down, and bring your hands around to meet your feet. Hang forward, relaxing your head, shoulders and spine. Hold the position for 10 full breaths. Inhale slowly to come up.

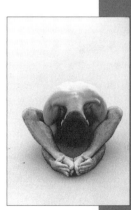

Complete this sequence with Preparation *Salamba Sarvangasana* (Chapter 5), Alternate-nostril breathing (Chapter 2) and *Savasana* B (Chapter 4).

pen your

eart and

ur mind with

ostures to

ease

motions,

mulate free

d easy

xpression

d enhance

getherness.

Intimacy and sharing

Reaching out for the touch, support, advice and love of others reminds us that we are a part of the whole – that we are not alone. Yoga means union and we can accentuate our joining by sharing our practice with a friend. Be creative with your practice and explore the joy of sharing. Communicate clearly with your partner in each posture to make sure it feels correct and to avoid overstretching.

Begin with Meditation while sitting back to back (Chapter 3), *Surya Namaskar* A (Chapter 6) and *Surya Namaskar* B (Chapter 6).

1. PARIGHASANA WITH A PARTNER – GATE POSE

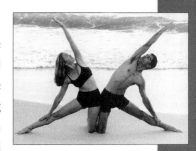

In this pose, one partner leans to the right and the other to the left. Have the toes of your kneeling leg and hip touching. Kneel beside each other and place your hand on the outside hip. Exhale and extend your right (or left) leg out to the right (or left), keeping the foot in line with your hip. Place your right (or left) hand on your right (or left) leg, down toward the foot. Inhale and extend out from the waist, raising your left (or right) arm. Exhale and extend your arm over your head, the palm facing down. Tuck in your chin and look beyond your left (or right) hand. Hold for 5 breaths, release and change sides.

2. ADHO MULCHA SVANASANA WITH A PARTNER – ADJUSTMENT

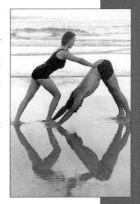

One person kneels with their hands on the ground below their shoulders, their feet hip-width apart. On the exhale, they tuck their toes under their feet and lift their hips and buttocks, releasing their heels to the ground. The partner places both hands on the sacrum and gently extends the partner's spine upward, keeping their own back straight and their front knee bent for support. Adjust each other in the pose for 5 to 10 full breaths.

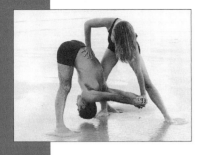

3. *PADOTTANASANA* III WITH A PARTNER – ADJUSTMENT

One person stands with their feet shoulder-width apart and their fingers interlocked behind their back. On the inhale, they extend up and out of the hips, and on the exhale, they release forward and down, keeping their legs locked straight and dropping their arms over their head toward the ground. The adjuster places one hand on the partner's lower back and the other on the partner's interlocked hands. Bending their knees, the adjuster supports the partner's forward movement by leaning into one leg. As the partner exhales, the adjuster can increase the pressure placed on the partner's hands, releasing them toward the ground. Hold this position for 10 breaths, release and swap positions.

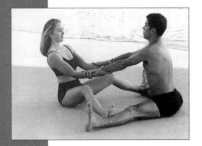

4. *KONASANA* WITH A PARTNER – ANGLE POSE

Both partners sit on the floor, backs straight and legs wide. The person being adjusted extends their arms out. The adjuster reaches and holds onto the partner's elbows, bends their own knees and places their heels into the partner's inner lower legs. As both exhale, the adjuster can spread the partner's legs wider by pushing with their heels; they can also draw the partner toward them by pulling their arms. The person being adjusted releases in the inner leg muscles. Adjust and hold each other in this pose for 10 deep, full breaths.

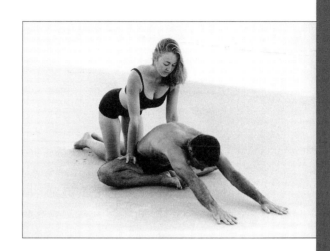

5. FORWARD *BADDHA KONASANA* WITH A PARTNER –
BOUND ANGLE POSE

One person sits with the soles of their feet together and hands interlocked around their feet. They inhale to lift out from the waist, and exhale to extend forward and release down. The adjuster kneels behind the partner, their hands resting on the partner's thighs or knees. Breathing together, as the partner inhales and lifts, the adjuster inhales; as the partner exhales and extends forward and releases down, the partner applies gentle pressure to their thighs or knees to open their hips. The adjuster can also apply pressure to the partner's lower back to assist them in lengthening forward and down. Hold for 10 deep, full breaths. Release and swap positions.

Sitting close together, complete the sequence with Cat curls (Chapter 6), Deep, full breathing (Chapter 2) sitting back to back and *Savasana* A (Chapter 4).

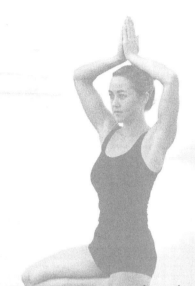

'hen it's time to

onfront

emanding and

allenging

sks,

oproach

em with a

ear mind and a

ove for detail

rough this

enewing

equence.

For mental clarity and concentration

Develop one-pointed focus with postures that cleanse and oxygenate the brain, giving you a "clean plate" to begin your day. Improve concentration levels on the job at hand with balancing inverted and backward-bending poses to energize you, sharpen your mind and activate your memory powers.

Begin with Forward hang (Chapter 5) Cat curls (Chapter 6) and *Surya Namaskar* C (Chapter 6).

1. VRKSASANA - TREE POSE

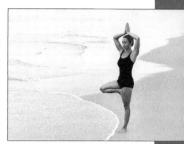

Begin in *Tadasana*, then bend your right leg, placing your right foot against your left thigh so it feels locked in. Move your right knee back to open your hip. Keep the muscles of your left leg activated and lifting. Center your bodyweight so that you aren't leaning on your standing leg too much. Place your hands in prayer position above your head. Roll your shoulders down and back to open your chest. Relax your facial muscles and gaze softly at a point in front at eye level. Hold for 5 full breaths. Exhale to release your leg and change sides.

2. ADHO MUKHA SVANASANA – DOWN FACE DOG POSE

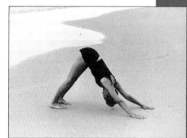

Kneel on the floor, extend your arms forward and step your feet back. Tucking your toes under, lift your hips and buttocks and straighten your legs, releasing your heels to the floor, hip-width apart. Soften your chest through your shoulders. Have a soft eye gaze in the direction of your feet. Hold for 5 to 10 breaths. Exhale as you release down, then rest.

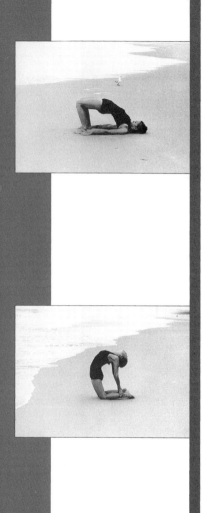

3. MINI BACKBEND

Lie on your back and bend your legs, placing your feet next to your buttocks, hip-width apart. Extend your arms alongside your body with the palms facing down. Exhale and slowly roll up off the floor, getting in touch with each vertebra as you do, first lifting your buttocks, then lower back, middle back and chest to form a backward arch. Keep your shoulders on the floor. Squeeze your buttocks together and lift your hips high. Hold for 5 breaths, release down, rest and repeat.

4. *USTRASANA* – CAMEL POSE

Kneel on the floor with your legs hip-width apart and hands on hips. Inhale and lift out from the waist and lower vertebrae. Exhale and slowly release your head back, bending your spine and pushing your hips forward. If you have the flexibility, rest your hands on your feet behind you; if not, place a chair behind you with a bolster on it and, as you descend, rest your elbows and arms on the bolster. Hold for 5 to 10 breaths. Inhale to come up, releasing one hand at a time for support.

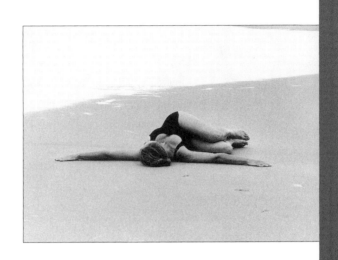

5. SPINAL ROLL

Lie on the floor on your back with your legs straight. Extend your arms out to the sides with the palms facing down. Inhale and bend your knees in to your chest. Exhale and turn your head to look beyond your left hand. Release your legs, still with knees bent, down to the floor on the right. Place your knees in close to your right armpit. Keep both shoulders flat to the floor. Hold for 5 deep, full breaths, releasing into the opening along your spine. Inhale to bring your legs back to center and repeat on the other side.

Complete the sequence with *Viparita Karani* (Chapter 5), Deep, full breathing (Chapter 2) and *Savasana* A (Chapter 4).

ng yourself

to the

resent by

cusing on all

e goodness

your life.

actice yoga to

vitalize

ur spirit and

go of the

st.

Depression

Depression is sometimes associated with lethargy and lack of inspiration. Get in touch with your body, breathe in some life-force and open up to what the present holds. Help overcome depression with dynamic postures that get you up and on the move again.

Begin with Forward hang (Chapter 5), *Surya Namaskar* A (Chapter 6) and *Surya Namaskar* C (Chapter 6).

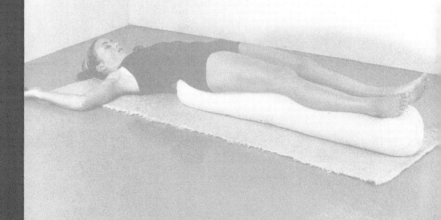

1. *SUPTA BADDHA KONASANA* LYING OVER A BOLSTER LENGTHWISE – SUPINE BOUND ANGLE POSE

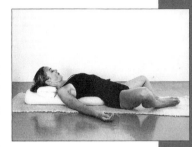

Sit with outstretched legs, a bolster or folded blankets extending lengthwise behind you. With your buttocks on the floor and your lower back touching the end of the bolster, exhale and lie back over the bolster, resting your head and upper back on it. Tuck in your chin and extend your arms to the sides. Bring the soles of your feet together and release your hips and knees to the floor. Focus on breathing fully and opening out your chest, lungs and heart. Rest in this position for 5 to 10 minutes.

2. *SETU BANDHA* SUPPORTED – BRIDGE POSE

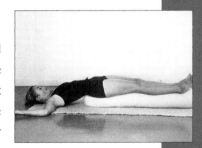

Lie on your back over a bolster or rolled blankets positioned lengthwise. Rest your head, shoulders and upper back on the floor, and allow your arms to relax above your head. This slight inversion position rests the heart, calms the mind and soothes the nervous system, helping relieve tension and headache. Close your eyes and rest in this pose for 10 minutes. To release out of the position, bend your knees and roll to one side.

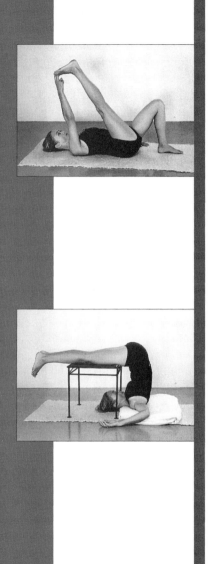

3. *SUPTA PADANGHUSTASANA* –
LYING DOWN LEG STRETCH POSE

Lie on your back, bend your left leg, and place the left foot on the floor toward your left hip. Inhale and raise your right leg, holding onto your foot with your right hand. Hold onto a belt around the foot if needed. Moving with the breath, release into the stretch in the hamstring and hip areas, by softening with each exhalation and allowing the leg to gently release forward and down. Hold for 5 to 10 breaths. Inhale to release and repeat on the other side.

4. SUPPORTED *HALASANA* – PLOUGH POSE

Place two or three folded blankets next to a chair with the folded edges facing inward. Lie with your back over the blankets, your shoulders on the edge of them and your head on the floor under the chair. Raise your legs up and over to rest the thighs along the seat of the chair. Relax your arms above your head on the floor. Hold for 5 to 10 minutes. To release, slowly raise your legs from the chair and return them slowly to the floor, resting before rolling to the side to come up.

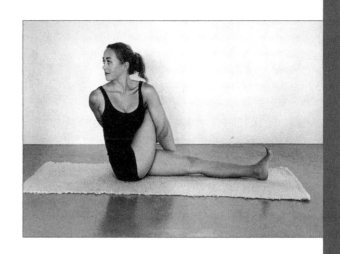

5. ARDHA MATSYENDRASANA VARIATION – HALF FISH LORD POSE

Sit with your legs extended out straight. Bend your right leg and place the right foot on the outside of your bent left knee. Inhale and place your left arm through your right knee. Inhale and turn to look over your right shoulder. Bring your right arm around and hold onto your right wrist with your left hand. Working in the pose, inhale to lift out from the waist, and exhale to twist and release deeper into the spine. After 5 full breaths, exhale to release and repeat on the opposite side.

Complete the sequence with Chair rest (Chapter 5), Deep, full breathing (Chapter 2) and *Savasana* B (Chapter 4).

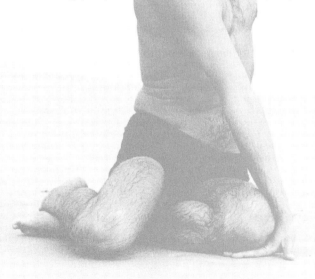

en your

art to

e-flowing,

ontaneous

pression,

ere there is no

ought, just

uth.

Open communication

When you're having trouble expressing yourself, overcome restrictions in the throat and open your chest area – where emotions are stored – with these postures. Allow your body to free your source of inner strength and speech. This sequence helps get you in touch with your heart and your truth, allowing you to be expressive and vocal and to believe in yourself.

Begin with Meditation (Chapter 3), Alternate-nostril breathing (Chapter 2) and *Surya Namaskar* A (Chapter 6).

1. BHARADVAJASANA – INDIAN SAGE POSE

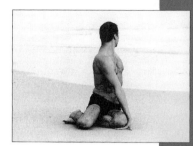

Sit on your buttocks, then bend your legs sideways so that your feet are next to your right hip. Place your left foot beneath your right foot. Inhale and come up and out from your waist, then twist your head and torso to the left. Place your right hand beside your left knee and your left hand around your back to hold on to your right hip. Turning to look over your left shoulder, rotate your left shoulder and elbow back. Hold for 5 breaths, release and change sides.

2. PADOTTANASANA III – FOOT-LEG EXTENSION POSE

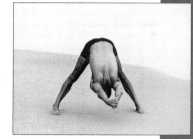

Stand with your feet about five feet apart. Interlock your fingers behind you. Inhale and raise your arms, extending up and out from your waist. Exhale and bend at your hips, slowly bringing your arms over your head and your hands toward the ground. Lock your legs, lean forward into the balls of your feet and feel the stretch in your hamstrings. Soften your spine, head and neck, and release your shoulders. Hold for 5 to 10 even breaths through the nose. Inhale to come up.

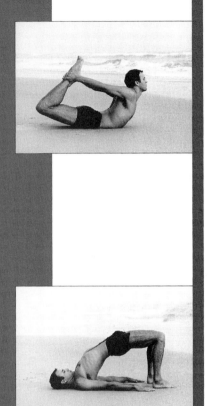

3. *DHANURASANA* – BOW POSE

Lie on your stomach, bend your knees, lifting your feet behind you in the air, and press your pubis to the floor. Inhale and bring your hands back to hold your ankles while raising your head and chest off the ground. Focus on drawing your head upward, your legs together, opening up your shoulders and lifting your chest. Look forward and lightly squeeze the buttocks. Hold for 5 full breaths. Exhale to release down, rest and repeat twice.

4. MINI BACKBEND

Lie on your back and bend your legs, placing your feet next to your buttocks, hip-width apart. Extend your arms alongside your body with the palms facing down. Exhale and slowly roll up off the floor, getting in touch with each vertebra as you do, first lifting your buttocks, then lower back, middle back and chest to form a backward arch. Keep your shoulders on the floor. Squeeze your buttocks together and lift your hips high. Hold for 5 breaths, release gently, rest and repeat.

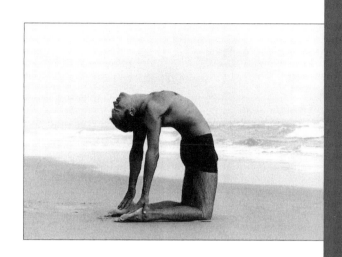

5. USTRASANA – CAMEL POSE

Kneel on the floor with your legs hip-width apart and hands on hips. Inhale and lift out from the waist and lower vertebrae. Exhale and slowly release your head back, bending your spine and pushing your hips forward. If you have the flexibility, rest your hands on your feet behind you; if not, place a chair behind you with a bolster on it and, as you descend, rest your elbows and arms on the bolster. Hold for 5 to 10 breaths. Inhale to come up, releasing one hand at a time for support.

Complete this sequence with East-west sequence (Chapter 6), Deep, full breathing (Chapter 2) and *Savasana* B (Chapter 4).

lease your

ine to discover

ourst of new

ergy that will

lp lift your

pirits and

ercome

dness.

Sadness and grief

Allow yourself to go through times of trauma, sadness, death and grief with love and understanding – from yourself. Create a nurturing space and spend time there, breathing deeply. Heal naturally with postures to release the spine, giving birth to a source of new energy and life.

Begin with Chair rest (Chapter 5), Deep, full breathing (Chapter 2) and East-west sequence (Chapter 6).

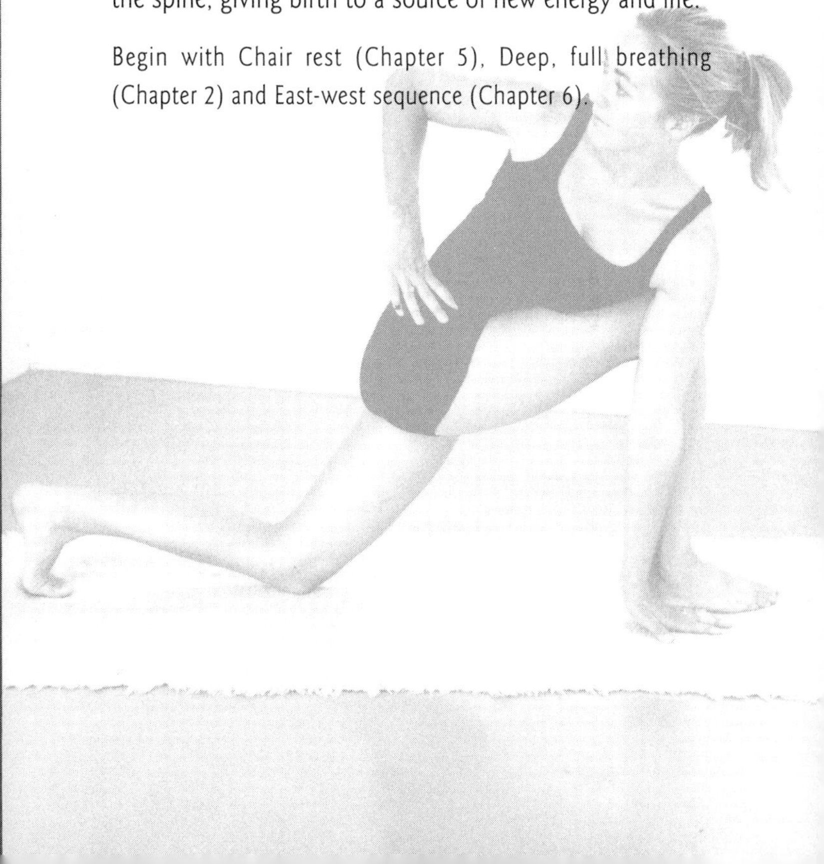

1. URDHVA MUKHA SVANASANA – UP FACE DOG POSE

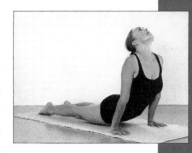

Lie on your stomach with your arms bent and the palms of your hands on the floor beside your shoulders and your legs extending away, with the tops of your feet on the floor. Inhale and raise your head, torso and hips off the floor. Roll your shoulders back to open up your chest. Keep your legs and arms locked. Focus forward or gently drop your head back. Hold for 10 deep, full breaths, expanding the chest fully. Exhale to release down and rest.

2. GOMUKHASANA – COW HEAD POSE

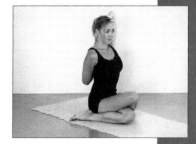

Kneel with your hands on the floor. Lean forward and cross your right leg over your left. Spread your feet away from your hips and sit between them on the floor. With your buttocks releasing down, bring your feet closer to your hips. Inhale and raise your left arm, bending your elbow and placing the palm of your hand down your back behind your head. Bring your right arm behind your back and interlock the fingers of both hands. Draw your left elbow away from your head. With each exhalation, focus on releasing deeper into the shoulders and hips. Hold for 5 breaths, release and repeat on other side.

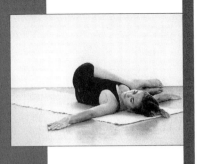

3. SPINAL ROLL

Lie on the floor on your back with your legs straight. Extend your arms out to the sides with the palms facing down. Inhale and bend your knees in to your chest. Exhale and turn your head to look beyond your left hand. Exhale and release your legs, still with knees bent, down to the floor on the right. Place your knees in close to your right armpit. Keep both shoulders flat on the floor. Hold for 5 deep, full breaths, releasing into the opening along your spine. Inhale to bring your legs back to center and repeat on the other side.

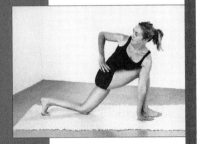

4. *PARIVRTTA PARSVAKONASANA* VARIATION –
REVOLVED SIDEWAYS ANGLE POSE

From a standing position, step your right foot forward about five feet and, squaring your hips to the front, lunge the right leg forward into a right angle. Rest your left knee on the floor. Inhale and raise your left arm. Exhale and turn to look over your right shoulder while placing your left hand on the floor beside your right foot. Rest your right hand on your right hip. Working with the breath, inhale to lift out from your waist, then exhale to twist further to the right. Hold for 5 breaths. Inhale to release out of the pose and change sides.

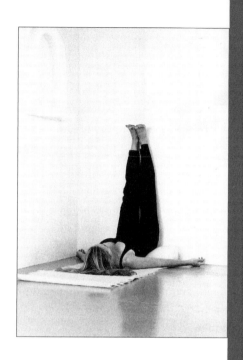

5. *VIPARITA KARANI* – INVERTED PRACTICE

Place a bolster or some folded blankets next to a wall. Lie with your legs up the wall, your hips and pelvis elevated on the bolster so that they are higher than your heart. Relax your upper back, shoulders, neck and head on the floor, and relax your arms, open on the floor to your sides or above your head, to open the chest and allow deep, full breathing. Rest in this gentle, relaxed, inverted position for 5 to 10 minutes.

Complete this sequence with Supported *Halasana* (Chapter 5), Deep, full breathing (Chapter 2) and *Savasana* B (Chapter 4).

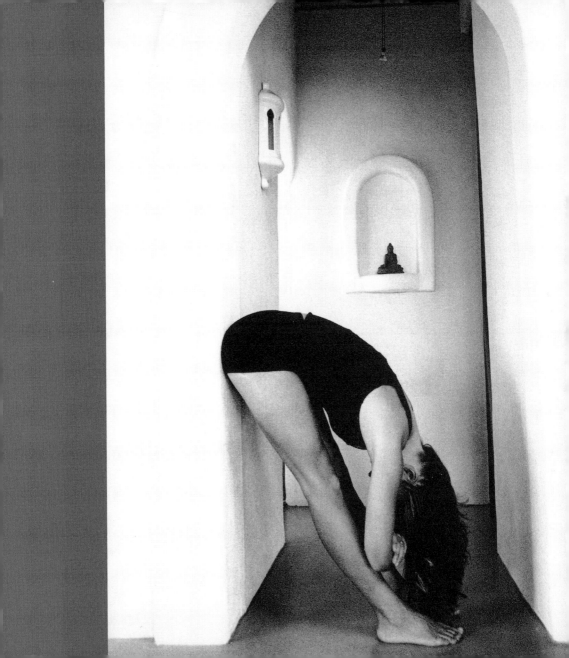

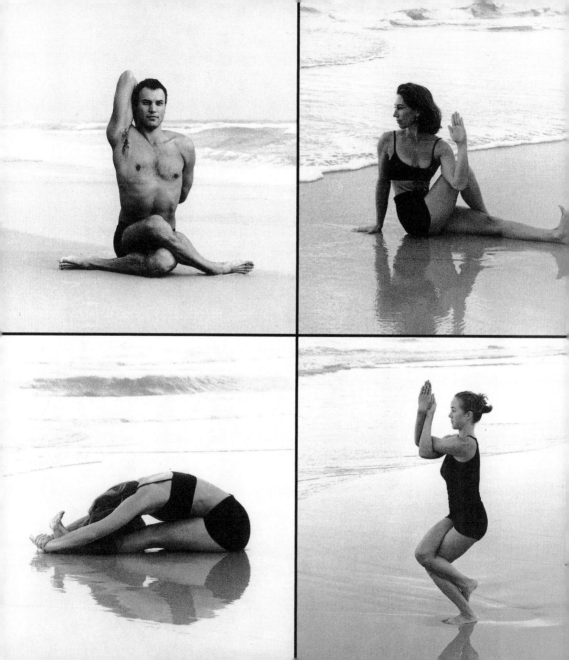

Body focus

Our physical body is one of our greatest teachers. You can learn a lot about yourself by observing your body, posture and the way you move.

The postures, or *asanas*, affect us on all levels: physically, mentally, emotionally and spiritually, making the physical journey a holistic one.

The balancing or homeostasic benefits of yoga affect people in different ways. While all postures strengthen and stretch the body, they also target specific internal systems such as the nervous, respiratory or hormonal systems, creating not only inner balance but also harmony and health.

When using postures to strengthen weak areas and stretch tight muscles, we naturally become aware of the subtler layers in our bodies. This understanding of our inner systems is one of the benefits of yoga practice, developing not only strength and flexibility but also self-awareness.

When in a posture, be aware of how it is affecting your body and your posture — notice where your body is asking you to contract and where to let go. Get in touch with your spine and aim to maintain balance on both your right and left side. Be sure that your mental state is calm and focused and that you are not straining or pushing. Maintain breath awareness, developing rhythmic breathing that is smooth and unrestricted.

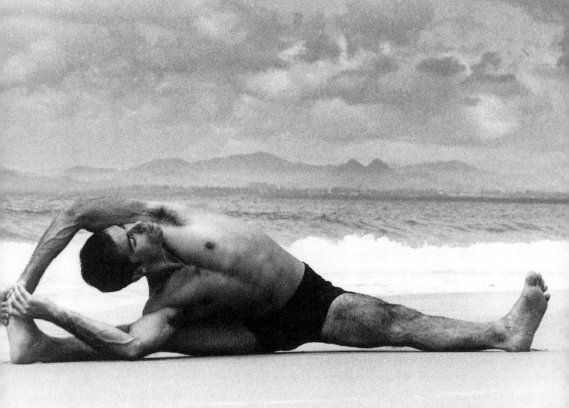

Creating balance

Release stiff joints

Keeping our joints mobile and their movement fluid requires exercise and maintaining good circulation. The joints are the hinges of our limbs and extremities, and if stiff or malnourished can cause movement-related aches and pains. Prevent degeneration by keeping your joints mobile with opening, cleansing and nourishing postures.

Begin with Deep, full breathing (Chapter 2), *Surya Namaskar* A (Chapter 6) and *Surya Namaskar* B (Chapter 6).

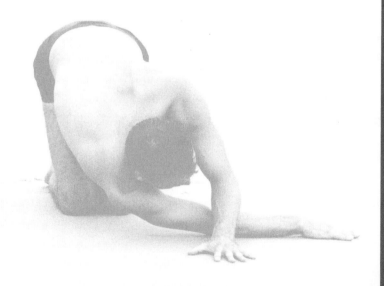

Yoga postures cleanse and renew the joints by bringing blood to the area to promote healthy synovial fluid, improve joint elasticity and strengthen the supporting ligaments.

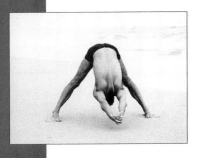

I. PADOTTANASANA III –
FOOT-LEG EXTENSION POSE

Stand with your feet about five feet apart. Interlock your fingers behind you. Inhale and raise your arms, extending up and out from your waist. Exhale and bend at your hips, slowly bringing your arms over your head and your hands toward the ground. Lock your legs, lean forward into the balls of your feet and feel the opening in the backs of your legs. Relax your spine, head and neck toward the floor, release your shoulders. Hold for 5 to 10 even breaths through the nose. Inhale to come up.

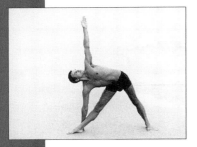

2. TRIKONSANA – TRIANGLE POSE

Stand with your feet about four feet apart. Turn your right foot out 90 degrees and the left foot in 45 degrees. Extend your arms out to the sides at shoulder height. Inhale and lengthen your right arm and the right side of your torso over to the right. Exhale and place your right hand onto your right ankle or the floor. Tuck your chin in, extend your left arm up and turn to look beyond the fingertips of your left hand. Keep the muscles of your legs and arms activated and the left hip opening. Inhale to release and bring yourself up. Exhale to turn and repeat on the other side.

3. GOMUKHASANA – COW HEAD POSE

Kneel with your hands on the floor. Lean forward and cross your right leg over your left. Spread your feet away from your hips and sit between them on the floor. With your buttocks releasing down, bring your feet closer to your hips. Inhale and raise your right arm, bending your elbow and placing the palm of your hand down your back behind your head. Bring your left arm behind your back and interlock the fingers. Draw your right elbow back away from your head. With each exhalation, focus on releasing deeper into the shoulders and hips. Hold for 5 breaths, release and repeat on other side.

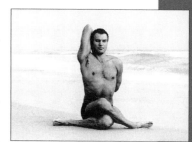

4. CAT SHOULDER STRETCH

Kneel on your hands and knees. Drop your right shoulder to the floor and, turning your head to look over your left shoulder, place your right arm under the left, reaching out the left. Feel the stretch in your right shoulder. Hold for 5 breaths, release and repeat with the left arm.

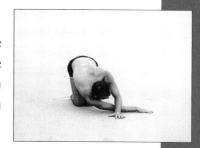

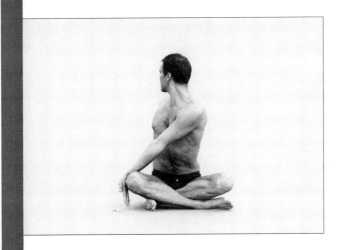

5. *SUKHASANA* TWIST – HAPPY TWIST POSE

Sit in an easy cross-legged position. With your back straight, place your left hand onto your right knee and your right hand behind you on the floor. Inhale to lift out from your waist, and exhale to twist and look over your right shoulder. Inhale to lift and exhale to twist for 5 breaths. Exhale and return to the center, then twist to the left side. Focus on releasing tension from your shoulders and hips with each exhalation. After 5 breaths, release, and come back to center.

Complete this sequence with *Viparita Karani* (Chapter 5), Cat curls (Chapter 6) and *Savasana* A (Chapter 4).

Release the spine and back muscles

Bring some life back into your spine with postures to loosen the vertebrae and release tension from the whole spine. When walking or sitting, keep your spine erect and focus on the elongation and separation of the vertebrae.

Begin with Deep, full breathing (Chapter 2), Cat curls (Chapter 6) and *Surya Namaskar* B (Chapter 6).

Focus on **elongating** and flexing the spine, promoting **tallness** and good posture.

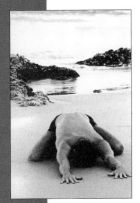

1. FORWARD REST

Kneel on the floor. Bring your big toes together and move your knees apart. Sit back on your buttocks, between the heels and on the soles of your feet. Inhale and walk your hands forward along the floor, lengthening your spine, and rest your forehead (third eye) to the floor. Keep your buttocks back at your heels and keep your arms extended forward to create a two-way stretch along the spine. Hold for 10 breaths. Inhale to come up.

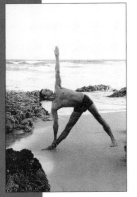

2. *TRIKONASANA* – TRIANGLE POSE

Stand with your feet about four feet apart. Turn your right foot out 90 degrees and the left foot in 45 degrees. Extend your arms out to the sides at shoulder height. Inhale and lengthen your right arm and the right side of your torso over to the right. Exhale and place your right hand onto your right ankle. Tuck your chin in, extend your left arm up and turn to look beyond the fingertips of your left hand. Keep the muscles of your legs and arms activated and the left hip opening. Inhale to release and bring yourself up. Exhale to turn and repeat on the other side.

3. CAT SHOULDER STRETCH

Kneel on your hands and knees. Drop your right shoulder to the floor and, turning your head to look over your left shoulder, place your right arm under the left, reaching out the left. Feel the stretch in your right shoulder. Hold for 5 breaths, release and repeat with the left arm.

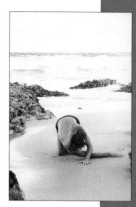

4. DHANURASANA – BOW POSE

Lie on your stomach, bend your knees, lifting your feet behind you in the air, and press your pubis to the floor. Inhale and bring your hands back to hold your ankles while raising your head and chest off the ground. Focus on drawing your head upward, your knees together, opening up your shoulders and lifting your chest. Look forward and lightly squeeze the buttocks. Hold for 5 full breaths. Exhale to release down, rest and repeat twice.

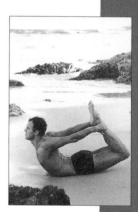

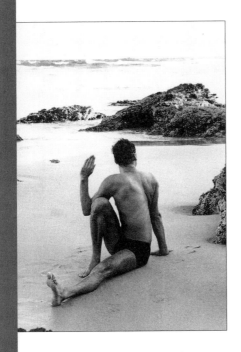

5. *MARICYASANA* TWIST – INDIAN SAGE POSE

Sit with your legs outstretched and bend your right leg, placing your foot on the floor near your groin so that your thigh is touching your abdomen. Place your right hand on the floor behind your right hip. Lock your left arm in front of your right knee. Inhale and lift up from your hips, thinning your waist. Exhale and twist to look over your right shoulder. Keep your left leg straight in front and the muscles activated. Release into the twist for 5 breaths. Release, come back to center, and repeat on the other side.

Complete the sequence with *Halasana* (Chapter 5), Meditation (Chapter 3) and *Savasana* C (Chapter 4).

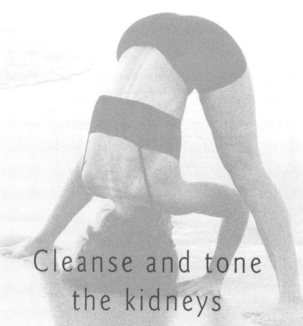

Cleanse and tone the kidneys

The kidneys are a main cleansing organ of the body. Overworking these vital waste-removers can result in fatigue, lethargy and lack of enthusiasm. Keeping your kidneys happy requires regular exercise and a healthy diet. Strengthen, tone and cleanse your kidneys often with this yoga sequence.

Begin with Deep, full breathing (Chapter 2), *Surya Namaskar* B (Chapter 6) and *Surya Namaskar* C (Chapter 6).

Help **overcome** kidney problems with postures to clean and **stimulate** – especially **therapeutic** after a night of indulgence.

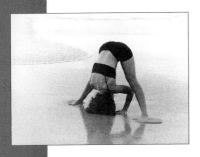

I. *PADOTTANASANA* I – FOOT-LEG EXTENSION POSE

Stand with your feet about five feet apart and your hands on your hips. Inhale and extend up and out from your waist. Exhale and slowly extend all the way forward and down, placing the palms of your hands on the floor between your feet. Activate and contract your front leg muscles, and lean forward into the balls of your feet, stretching the backs of your legs. Soften your spine, head and neck, keeping your shoulders lifted. Hold 5 to 10 even breaths through the nose. Inhale to come up.

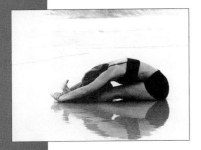

2. *PASCIMOTTANASANA* – BACK EXTENSION POSE

Sit with your legs extended straight out in front and activated. Lift the fleshy part of your buttocks, roll onto your sitting bones, and tilt your pelvis forward. Inhale to lift and extend your pubis, stomach and chest. Exhale to release down and lie over your outstretched legs. Keep both legs locked and the toes working back toward your head, and your eye focus toward your feet. Hold for 5 to 10 deep, full breaths. Inhale to release. Use a belt around your feet and stay sitting upright if you can't rest forward.

3. *ARDHA MATSYENDRASANA* VARIATION – HALF FISH LORD POSE

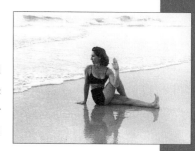

Sit with your legs extended out straight. Bend your right leg and place the right foot on the outside of your straight left knee. Place your left arm over your right knee. Inhale and turn to look over your right shoulder, placing your right hand behind you on the ground for support. Working in the pose, inhale to lift out from the waist, and exhale to twist and release deeper into the spine. After 5 full breaths, exhale to release and repeat on the opposite side.

4. *JATHARA PARIVARTANASANA* – STOMACH TURN POSE

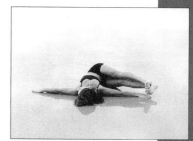

Lie on your back with your arms extended out to the sides, palms facing downward. Exhale and raise your legs to create a 90-degree angle to your torso. Keeping your back flat on the floor, turn your head to the left, lift your hips slightly to the left and slowly release your legs down to the right. If possible hover your feet beside your right hand without touching the floor, otherwise rest your legs on the floor. Hold for 5 breaths, then inhale your legs up to center and repeat on the other side. Repeat the full sequence twice.

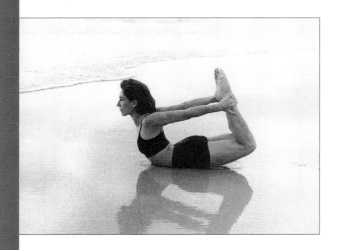

5. *DHANURASANA* – BOW POSE

Lie on your stomach, bend your knees, lifting your feet behind you in the air, and press your pubis to the floor. Inhale and bring your hands back to hold your ankles while raising your head and chest off the ground. Focus on drawing your head upward, your knees together, opening up your shoulders and lifting your chest. Look forward and lightly squeeze the buttocks. Hold for 5 full breaths. Exhale to release down, rest and repeat twice.

Complete this sequence with East-west sequence (Chapter 6), Supported *Halasana* (Chapter 5) and *Savasana* D (Chapter 4).

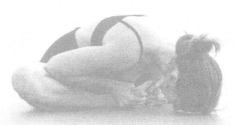

Cleansing and toning the sexual organs

Strong, healthy sexual organs and glands enhance energy on all levels. Open up the pelvic region with these postures to encourage nutritive circulation to the reproductive organs, regulate menstrual flow and relieve pelvic congestion.

Begin with *Viparita Karani* (Chapter 5), Cat curls (Chapter 6) and *Surya Namaskar* B (Chapter 6).

Get in touch with your **life-giving** source through this strengthening and **nourishing** sequence.

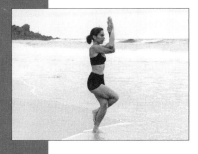

1. GARUDASANA – EAGLE POSE

Stand with your feet together. Bend your knees and cross your right leg over the left, tucking your right foot behind your left ankle. Keeping your knees bent, raise your arms to shoulder height. Bend your forearms up to create a 90-degree angle. Cross your left arm over the right, bringing the left palm around to meet the right palm and stretching your hands and wrists. Keep your forearms moving away from your head and your gaze forward. Hold for 5 breaths then repeat on the other side.

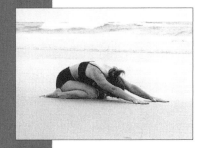

2. FORWARD VIRASANA – HERO POSE

Sit with your buttocks on your heels, then slide your heels out to the sides so your buttocks release to the floor between them. Draw your knees in together. Sit upright, extending the spine. Inhale and raise your arms. Exhale and extend your torso forward, lying along the floor with your arms extending forward. Keep your buttocks down and focus on releasing in the hips and groin. Hold for 10 breaths. Exhale to release up.

3. FORWARD *BADDHA KONASANA* –
BOUND ANGLE POSE

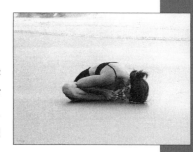

Sit with the soles of your feet together. Let your knees relax to the floor and the muscles around the hips soften. Interlock your fingers around your toes. Inhale and lift out from your lower back. Exhale to lift up through the front of your body, stomach and chest, then extend forward and down to rest first your abdomen, then your chest, then your forehead to the floor. Breathe into the opening around your hips, softening with each exhalation. Hold for 10 deep, full breaths.

4. *UPAVISTA KONASANA* – SEATED ANGLE POSE

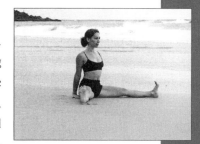

Sit on the floor with your legs wide apart and toes pointing up. Activate your leg muscles and focus on softening and breathing into the inner leg. Keep your knees in line with your feet. Place your hands on the floor behind you, your fingers facing forward, and use your arms to support you as you tilt your pelvis forward slightly and open your inner leg and groin softly, without over-stretching. Soften here for 10 deep, full breaths.

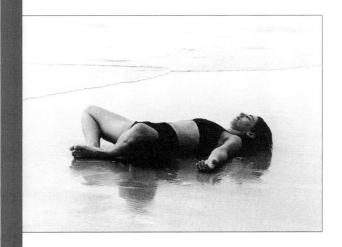

5. SUPTA BADDHA KONASANA – SUPINE BOUND ANGLE POSE

Lie flat on your back. Bend your knees and bring the soles of your feet together, then let your feet splay open and drop your knees to the floor, releasing your hips. Extend your arms out to your sides away from your body, palms facing upward. Close your eyes and breathe fully, releasing the hips with each exhalation. Rest for as long as comfortable; 5 to 10 minutes is effective.

Complete this sequence with *Sarvangasana* (Chapter 5), Alternate-nostril breathing (Chapter 2) and *Savasana* D (Chapter 4).

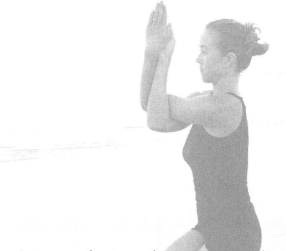

Stretch and strengthen the legs, feet and ankles

Your legs and feet are your foundation. A strong and stable lower body allows you to be free and mobile in your upper body. Strengthen, stretch and balance your base with the following sequence of postures.

Begin with Deep, full breathing (Chapter 2), *Surya Namaskar* A (Chapter 6) and *Surya Namaskar* B (Chapter 6).

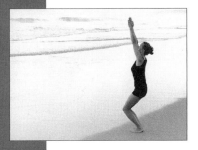

1. *UTKATASANA* – POWERFUL POSE

Stand with your feet together. Inhale and raise your arms above your head, bringing your palms together. Exhale and bend your knees, keeping your heels down. Lock your elbows and extend your spine out from your hips. Breathe fully into your chest, lifting and expanding your rib cage. Tuck your buttocks under and keep your back straight. Hold for 5 to 10 deep, full breaths. Exhale to release.

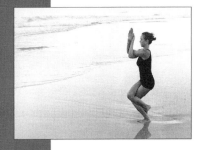

2. *GARUDASANA* – EAGLE POSE

Stand with your feet together. Bend your knees and cross your right leg over the left, tucking your right foot behind your left ankle. Keeping your knees bent, raise your arms to shoulder height. Bend your forearms up to create a 90-degree angle. Cross your left arm over the right, bringing the left palm around to meet the right palm and stretching your hands and wrists. Keep your forearms moving away from your head and your gaze forward. Hold for 5 breaths then repeat on the other side.

3. ADHO MUKHA SVANASANA –
DOWN FACE DOG POSE

Kneel on the floor, extend your arms forward and step your feet back. Tucking your toes under, lift your hips and buttocks and straighten your legs, releasing your heels to the floor. Soften your chest through your shoulders. Have a soft eye gaze in the direction of your feet. Hold for 5 to 10 breaths. Exhale as you release down, then rest.

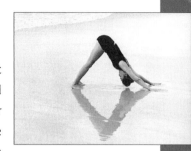

4. SUPTA PADAGHUSTASANA –
LYING DOWN STRETCH LEG POSE

Lie on your back, bend your left leg, and place the left foot on the floor toward your left hip. Inhale and raise your right leg, holding onto your foot with your right hand. Loop a belt over your foot to hold onto if you can't reach. Moving with the breath, release into the stretch in the hamstring and hip areas by softening with each exhalation and allowing the leg to gently release forward and down. Hold for 5 to 10 breaths. Inhale to release and repeat on the other side.

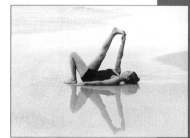

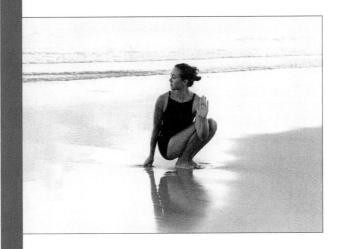

5. *PASASANA* VARIATION – NOOSE POSE

Squat with your feet together. Exhale, turn to the right and place your right hand on the floor behind you. Bend your left arm and lock it over your right knee. Maintain your balance, stretching deep into your ankles by leaning forward into the front of your feet. Keep your head turned to the right. Hold for 5 breaths. Exhale to release and change sides. Rest your heels on a blanket if needed.

Complete this sequence with East-west sequence (Chapter 6), Meditation (Chapter 3) and *Savasana* C (Chapter 4).

Abdominal toning

The various muscles of the midriff form a protective wall around your internal abdominal organs. These muscles also work in unison with your back muscles to hold your spine erect. Practice the following postures to tone and strengthen your core center.

Begin with Alternate-nostril breathing (Chapter 2), *Surya Namaskar* A (Chapter 6) and *Surya Namaskar* B (Chapter 6).

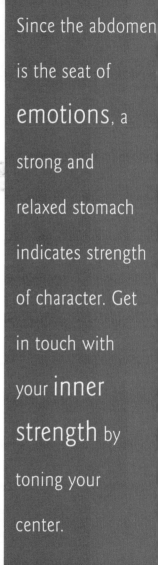

Since the abdomen is the seat of **emotions**, a strong and relaxed stomach indicates strength of character. Get in touch with your **inner strength** by toning your center.

1. LEG LIFT I

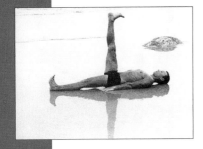

Lie flat on the floor with your legs extended. Exhale to slowly raise your right leg to 90 degrees. Hold for 5 breaths, then inhale to release the leg to the floor. Exhale to slowly raise your left leg to 90 degrees. Hold for 5 breaths, then inhale to release it to the floor. Repeat the full cycle 3 times.

2. LEG LIFT II

Lie flat on the floor with your legs extended. Place your palms face down beside your buttocks. Exhale to slowly raise both legs together to 90 degrees. Hold for 5 breaths, then inhale to slowly release your legs to just a few inches above the floor. Exhale to raise your legs. Hold. Inhale to release. Do this 3 to 5 times, then rest. Keep your legs bent if needed.

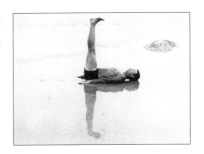

3. JATHARA PARIVARTANASANA – STOMACH TURN POSE

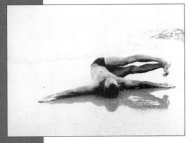

Lie on your back with your arms extended out and palms facing down. Exhale and raise your legs to 90 degrees to your torso. Keep your back flat on the floor and your head centered, lock your legs, lift your hips slightly to the left and slowly release your legs to the right. Hover your feet beside your right hand or rest your legs down. Hold for 5 breaths, then inhale, lifting your legs up to center and repeat on the other side. Repeat twice.

4. SALABHASANA – LOCUST POSE

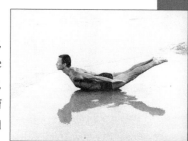

Lie on your stomach and place your arms alongside your body, your palms facing upward. Rest your forehead on the floor. Inhale to raise your head, chest, arms, shoulders and legs off the floor, activating and strengthening your entire back; only the front of your torso and hips are in contact with the floor. Focus forward and hold the position for 10 even breaths. Inhale to release down, rest and repeat twice.

5. ARDHA MATSYENDRASANA VARIATION – HALF FISH LORD POSE

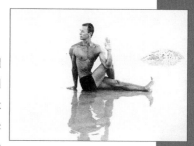

Sit with your legs extended out straight. Bend your right leg and place the right foot on the outside of your left knee. Inhale and place your left arm over your right knee. Inhale and turn to look over your right shoulder, placing your right hand behind you on the ground for support. Working in the pose, inhale to lift out from the waist, and exhale to twist and release deeper into the spine. After 5 full breaths, exhale to release and repeat on the opposite side.

Complete this sequence with the East-west sequence (Chapter 6), Deep, full breathing (Chapter 2) and *Savasana* C (Chapter 4).

proactive

out your

oblems, and

lp release

nsion with

retching

d deep

reathing.

Release neck and shoulder tension

Many people store tension and stress in their neck and shoulders. Regular massage will help to release and relax these muscles, as will these yoga postures. If you often complain of tightness in the neck and shoulders, practice these postures regularly and feel tension melt away with the breath.

Begin with Deep, full breathing (Chapter 2), Cat curls (Chapter 6) and Forward hang (Chapter 5).

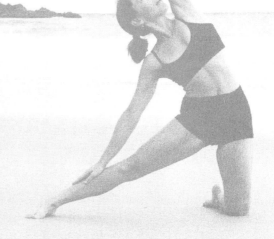

1. *PADOTTANASANA* III –
FOOT-LEG EXTENSION POSE

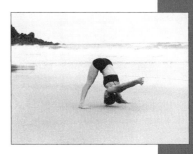

Stand with your feet about five feet apart. Interlock your fingers behind you. Inhale and raise your arms, extending up and out from your waist. Exhale and bend at your hips, slowly bringing your arms over your head and your hands toward the ground. Lock your legs, lean forward into the balls of your feet and feel the stretch in the backs of your legs. Relax your spine, head and neck toward the floor, releasing your shoulders. Hold for 5 to 10 even breaths through the nose. Inhale to come up.

2. CAT SHOULDER STRETCH

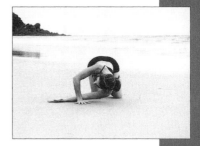

Kneel on your hands and knees. Drop your left shoulder to the floor and, turning your head to look over your right shoulder, place your left arm under the right, reaching out the left. Feel the stretch in your left shoulder. Hold for 5 breaths, release and repeat with the right arm.

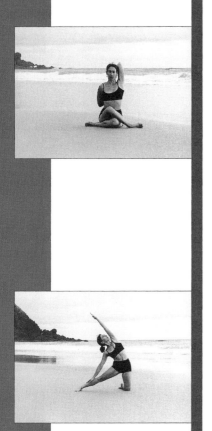

3. GOMUKHASANA – COW HEAD POSE

Kneel with your hands on the floor. Lean forward and cross your right leg over your left. Spread your feet away from your hips and sit between them on the floor. With your buttocks releasing down, bring your feet closer to your hips. Inhale and raise your left arm, bending your elbow and placing the palm of your hand down. Bring your right arm behind your back and interlock the fingers. Draw your left elbow away from your head. Focus on releasing deeper into the shoulders and hips. Hold for 5 breaths, release and repeat on other side.

4. PARIGHASANA – GATE POSE

Kneel on the floor and place your hands on your hips. Exhale and extend your right leg out to the right, keeping the foot in line with your hip. Place your right hand on your right leg, down toward the foot. Inhale and extend out from the waist, raising your left arm. Exhale and extend your left arm over your head, the palm facing down. Tuck in your chin and either look up to the left hand or to the floor. Keep the left hip above the left knee. Breathe into the side of your torso as you release in the stretch for 5 breaths. Inhale to release and repeat on the other side.

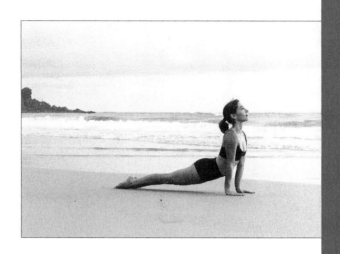

5. URDHVA MUKHA SVANASANA – UP FACE DOG POSE

Lie on your stomach with your arms bent and the palms of your hands on the floor beside your shoulders and your legs extending away, with the tops of your feet on the floor. Inhale and raise your head, torso and hips off the floor. Roll your shoulders back to open up your chest. Keep your legs and arms locked. Focus forward or gently drop your head back. Hold for 10 deep, full breaths, expanding the chest fully. Exhale to release down and rest.

Complete this sequence with *Halasana* (Chapter 6), Meditation (Chapter 3) and *Savasana* B (Chapter 4).

eeling

ninspired or

thargic?

et your body

efresh your

rain with these

leansing and

timulating

ostures.

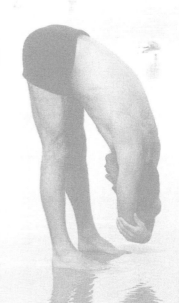

Stimulate the brain

Next time you feel the need to reach for an artificial stimulant to stay alert and awake, try these naturally stimulating postures that activate the nervous system and stimulate circulation to the brain. You will feel clear, focused and refreshed.

Begin with Deep, full breathing (Chapter 2), East-west sequence (Chapter 6) and *Surya Namaskar* A (Chapter 6).

1. UTTANASANA – EXTENSION POSE

Stand with your feet hip-width apart and interlock your thumbs into the crease of the opposite elbow. Inhale to raise your arms above your head. Exhale to bend at the hips and release your upper body forward and down. Tuck your chin in and focus up to your navel. While breathing deeply and fully, relax your head, neck and shoulders, release your spine and stretch the backs of your legs. Hold for 10 breaths, then bend your knees, inhale and come up slowly.

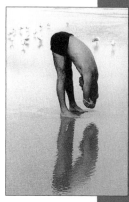

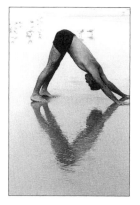

2. ADHO MUKHA SVANASANA – DOWN FACE DOG POSE

Kneel on the floor, extend your arms forward and step your feet back. Tucking your toes under, lift your hips and buttocks and straighten your legs, releasing your heels. Soften your chest through your shoulders. Have a soft eye gaze in the direction of your feet. Hold for 5 to 10 breaths. Exhale as you release down, then rest.

3. MATSYENDRASANA VARIATION – FISH POSE

Lie on your back with your arms at your sides. Inhale to raise your head and chest off the floor. Rest your head back, creating an arch in your back. Puff your chest forward, keeping your shoulders and arms on the floor and your legs straight. Hold for 10 breaths. Inhale to lift your head off the floor, exhale to tuck your chin into your chest and release your whole body to the floor.

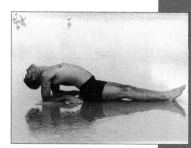

4. MINI BACKBEND

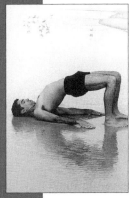

Lie on your back and bend your legs, placing your feet next to your buttocks, hip-width apart. Extend your arms alongside your body with the palms facing down. Exhale and slowly roll up off the floor, getting in touch with each vertebra as you do, first lifting your buttocks, then lower back, middle back and chest to form a backward arch. Keep your shoulders on the floor. Squeeze your buttocks together and lift your hips high. Hold for 5 breaths, release gently, rest and repeat.

5. SPINAL ROLL

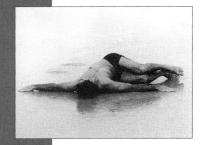

Lie on the floor on your back with your legs straight. Extend your arms out to the sides with the palms facing down. Inhale and bend your knees in to your chest and turn your head to face beyond your left hand. Exhale and release your bent legs down to the right, bringing your knees close to your right armpit. Keep both shoulders flat to the floor. Hold for 5 deep, full breaths, releasing into the opening along your spine. Inhale to bring your legs back to center and repeat on the other side.

Complete this sequence with Preparation *Salamba Sarvangasana* (Chapter 5), Alternate-nostril breathing (Chapter 2) and *Savasana* A (Chapter 4).

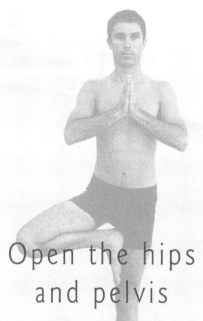

Open the hips and pelvis

Flexible, strong hips help to support your spine and make getting around easier. Keep your hip joints and muscles strong, supple and open with these strengthening and stretching postures, and enjoy the freedom this creates for the journey of life!

Begin with Deep, full breathing (Chapter 2), *Surya Namaskar* A (Chapter 6) and *Surya Namaskar* B (Chapter 6).

Get in touch with the feeling of **freedom** that supple hips and pelvic muscles can create with these stretching and **opening** postures.

1. *VRKSASANA* – TREE POSE

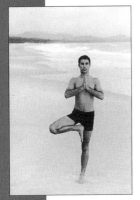

Begin in *Tadasana*, then bend your right leg, placing your right foot against your left thigh so it feels locked in. Move your right knee back to open your hip. Keep the muscles of your left leg activated. Center your bodyweight. Place your hands in prayer position in front of your heart. Roll your shoulders down and back, relax your face and gaze forward. Hold for 5 full breaths. Exhale to release your leg and change sides.

2. *GARUDASANA* – EAGLE POSE

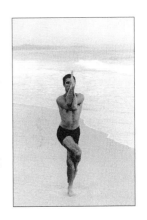

Stand with your feet together. Bend your knees and cross your right leg over the left, tucking your right foot behind your left ankle. Keeping your knees bent, raise your arms to shoulder height. Bend your forearms 90 degrees. Cross your left arm over the right, bringing the left palm around to meet the right palm and stretching your forearms away from your head.

3. HIP STRETCH

Sit on the floor with your legs outstretched. Bend your right knee and rest it on the floor away from your hips. Bring your left foot to rest on the right knee, and the left knee to rest on your right foot. Inhale and, with your hands on the floor in front of you, exhale and lean forward, releasing the left knee down. Hold for a few breaths and repeat on the other side.

4. GOMUKHASANA – COW HEAD POSE

Kneel with your hands on the floor. Lean forward and cross your right leg over your left. Sit back on your left heel. With your buttocks releasing down, bring your right foot closer to your left hip. Inhale and raise your left arm, bending your elbow and placing the palm of your hand down your back behind your head. Bring your right arm behind your back and interlock the fingers of both hands. Draw your left elbow away from your head. With each exhalation, focus on releasing deeper into the shoulders and hips. Hold for 5 breaths, release and repeat on other side.

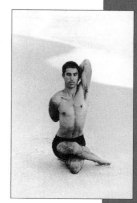

5. SUPTA BADDHA KONASANA – SUPINE BOUND ANGLE POSE

Lie flat on your back. Bend your knees and bring the soles of your feet together, then let your feet splay open and drop your knees to the floor, releasing your hips. Rest your arms out to your sides away from your body, releasing the hips with the exhalation breath. Close your eyes and breathe fully. 5 to 10 minutes is effective.

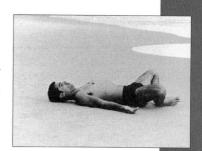

Complete this sequence with Cat curls (Chapter 6), Meditation (Chapter 3) and *Savasana* D (Chapter 4).

nlock your

pirit and free

ur heart and

evelop full

reathing

ith these

eeply

herapeutic

ostures that

evelop

penness of

ody and mind.

Open the chest, heart and lungs

Good posture and an open chest are signs of a confident, open and healthy person. Keep your heart open to love and life with these postures that stretch your chest muscles and stimulate circulation.

Begin with Cat curls (Chapter 6), Alternate-nostril breathing (Chapter 2) and *Surya Namaskar* B (Chapter 6).

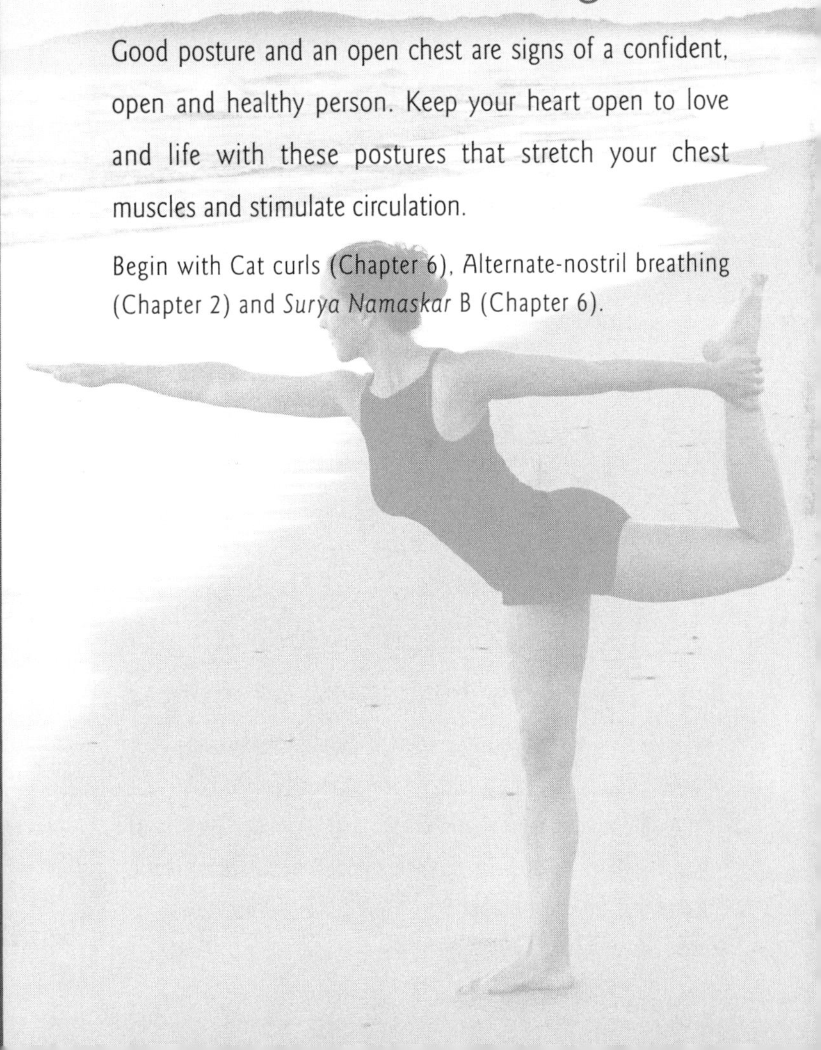

1. *NATARAJASANA* VARIATION – DANCER'S POSE

Stand with your feet hip-width apart. Bend your right leg behind you and hold onto the right ankle with your right hand. Extend your left arm forward and, leaning forward into your standing leg, raise your right leg up and back, away from your body. Soften your lower back area. Maintain eye focus straight ahead. Focus on releasing within the spine and the ankle, knee, hip and shoulder joints. Hold for 5 breaths, release and repeat on the opposite side.

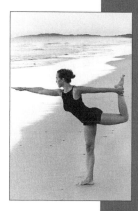

2. *NAMASTE* BEHIND THE BACK

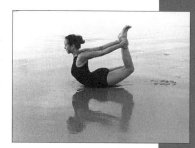

While standing or sitting, reach behind your back and bring your hands into the *Namaste*, or prayer, position. Feel your shoulders and chest opening up and allow any tension and stiffness in your hands to release. Hold for 10 breaths. Practice this posture to release tension and promote correct breathing.

3. *DHANURASANA* – BOW POSE

Lie on your stomach, bend your knees, lift your feet and press your pubis to the floor. Inhale and bring your hands back to hold your ankles and raise your head and chest off the ground. Draw your knees together, open your shoulders and lift your chest. Look forward and squeeze the buttocks. Hold for 5 breaths. Exhale to release down, rest and repeat twice.

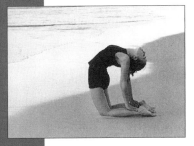

4. *USTRASANA* – CAMEL POSE

Kneel on the floor with your legs hip-width apart and hands on hips. Inhale and lift out from the waist and lower vertebrae. Exhale and slowly release your head back, bending your spine and pushing your hips forward. If you have the flexibility, rest your hands on your feet behind you; if not, place a chair behind you with a bolster on it and, as you descend, rest your elbows and arms on the bolster. Hold for 5 to 10 breaths. Inhale to come up, releasing one hand at a time for support.

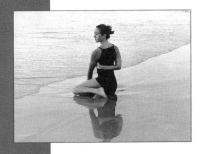

5. *BHARADVAJASANA* – INDIAN SAGE POSE

Sit on your buttocks, then bend your legs sideways so that your feet are next to your left hip. Place your left foot on top of your right foot. Inhale and come up and out from your waist, then twist your head and torso to the right. Place your left hand beside your right knee and wrap your right hand around your back to hold on to your left elbow or hip. Turning to look over your left shoulder, rotate your right shoulder and elbow back. Hold for 5 breaths, release and change sides.

Complete this sequence with East-west sequence (Chapter 6), Deep, full breathing (Chapter 2) and *Savasana* B (Chapter 4).

Index

About the author

Jessie Chapman is the author of *Yoga in Focus*. Jessie first discovered yoga in 1991 and was instantly hooked. She was inspired by the positive effect it had on her mental state, emotions and body. In yoga, she discovered a key to overcoming limiting beliefs and lifestyle habits, freeing her spirit and getting in touch with her potential in life. She explored many different styles of yoga and in 1997 completed the Yoga Arts Nine-Month Teacher Training Certificate Course. She has been teaching since. She aims to inspire beginners to yoga through the simplicity of its practice and its inspiring benefits. Jessie lives in Byron Bay, Australia, and is a columnist for *Pure* magazine.

About the photographer

Dhyan took the photographs for Jessie's first book, *Yoga in Focus*. He first discovered the joy of photography twenty years ago while traveling through South America. His "no fear," lighthearted and humorous approach to life has taken him to some unusual and beautiful places, enriching his life experiences, deepening his spiritual connection within and making him an enjoyable photographer to model for. Dhyan is based in Byron Bay and Bali, builds Indonesian-influenced houses, surfs, swims with the dolphins, hangs out with his gorgeous son Kai, gardens and travels.

Jessie also took some of the photos, re-igniting her passion for photography.

Acknowledgments

I give much gratitude to all the yoga teachers I have learned from for inspiring me with your experience, for openly sharing your knowledge and personal insights, and for teaching with passion. A big thanks to all the people who I have learned from as a teacher myself — people who shared their yoga experiences, people with injuries, headaches, overworked muscles from different sports and simply tight body parts — all greatly contributed to the creation of this book of sequences for specific purposes.

Many thanks to Dhyan for another great team effort and for all the gorgeous photos. Those many up-at-the-crack-of-dawn mornings, scouting the beaches for the cleanest set, the lowest tide and calmest seas, were all worth it! A special thank you to the yoga models who captured so beautifully the essence of the poses and made the book a joy to create: James Bahuth (jbahuth@hotmail.com), Pete Watkins (petewatkins@yahoo.com.au), Rachel Hull (rachelhull@hotmail.com), Mark Hill and myself (jessie_2481@yahoo.com). It was not always easy but the glorious sunrises made up for it all!

Printing the photos was an enormous task; thanks so much, John Derry, for your patience, generosity and expertise with the photography; we could not have finished this on time without you. Thank you, Mark Geritson, for your kindness and generosity with your dark room, and Rachel Hull for the loan of the yoga props.

Thanks, gorgeous Vibousha, for the loan of your beautiful house for the inside shots, again.

A special thank you to my mother, CC, for your patience and support whenever needed and to my sister Judy, who motivates and inspires me, I love you both. To my friends and family, thanks for being there.

Thanks to all the HarperCollins publishing team who saw the book through to its completion, especially Helen Littleton for sharing my vision; Katie Mitchell for your creative eye and stunning layout and design; Veronica Miller and the editing team for your wonderful word work; and Helen Johnson. I really appreciate all your support and expertise, which made this book possible.

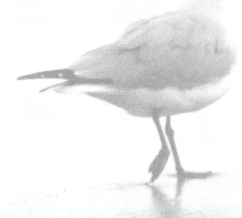

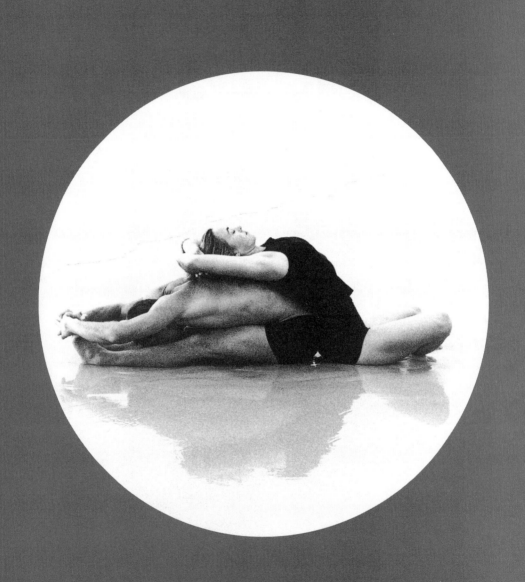